AYURVEDA

a historical perspective

Dr Ranganayakulu Ph.D.,
India

Pangea Publishers

Ayurveda
a historical perspective
2015

ranganayakulu@hotmail.com

Published by Amazon, USA for Pangea, India
Coverpage: a stone sculpture of Bodhi Tree, 15th c.
Ayuthaya. National Museum of Bankok, Thailand

Transliteration Scheme

ā	as in f**a**ther
bh	as in a**bh**or
c	as in chur**ch**
ch	as in **ch**ill
d	as in **th**at
ḍ	as in **d**rum
dh	as in **dh**arma
ḍh	as in re**dh**aired
gh	as in lo**gh**ut
ī	as in pol**i**ce
jh	as in he**dg**ehog
kh	as in in**kh**orn
m	as in **m**ap, ja**m**
ṃ	as in Sa**m**skruta
n	as in **n**ot, **n**ut, i**n**
ṇ	as in no**n**e
ṅ	as in si**n**g, ki**n**g
ñ	as in su**n**g
o	as in g**o**, st**o**ne
p	as in **p**ut, si**p**
ph	as in u**ph**ill
r	as in **r**ed, yea**r**
ṛ	as in me**rr**y, ma**r**ine
s	as in **s**aint, **s**in, hi**ss**
ś	as in **s**ure, **s**iva
ṣ	as in **sh**un, bu**sh**
t	as in ba**th**

ṭ	as in **tr**ue
th	as in **th**eatre
ṭh	as in an**th**ill

Index

Preface

I chose ayurveda as my career by chance. Having spent thirty years in the teaching and practice of ayurveda, I could not resist from writing this book. I do not intend just to narrate the story of ayurveda but to offer a critical view of its checkered past and its ambiguous role in today's public health.

Many ayurveda scholars in India regard ayurveda as a consistent, complete and scientific system of medicine and consider it as the *Indian* way of science! They believe in myriad mythological stories and divine origins of medicine. Ayurveda is believed to have been created in a flash of time, not evolved during the course of centuries. The treatises of ayurveda reflect its approach to health, its struggle to understand the disease process, its sincerity in finding therapies and its compromising attitude with incurable diseases. However, remember the saying of Jawaharlal Nehru, the first prime minister of India, 'learn all you can from the ancient systems of medicine and surgery but do not believe that the last word has been said a thousand years ago'.

Western medicine has overtaken ayurveda decades ago in terms of utility, popularity, acceptability and spread in India. The people of India take ayurveda as divine and ageless. A sore feeling haunts me that very few scholars in India are interested in the history of medicine. It is surprising that no university in India offers a course in the history of science and medicine to help physicians to dispel their ignorance. Besides, very few general historians in the universities of India are engaged in the history of science. There is a big gap in interdisciplinary studies here. The knowledge of medicine without history cannot have a human face.

I was first exposed to the writings of O.P. Jaggi, Kutumba Rao, Subba Reddy, Subbarayappa, P.V. Sharma and others. The writings of Filliozat, Julius Jolly, Henri Sigerest, Dominique Wujastyk, Kenneth Zysk, Maulenbeld and others gave me a new perspective on the history of medicine and ayurveda. It is the right time to examine the history of ayurveda to integrate it with other systems of medicine for optimal health care.

The purpose of this book is to explore the evolution of ideas in ayurveda and the rationality of those ideas. Now, the world looks at ayurveda with renewed interest. Many believe in the foundations of ayurveda as unfathomable and undisputable. I wish the prospective physicians and teachers of ayurveda in India to be saved from the fallacies that have been deliberately shoved onto the minds.

There are professors and specialists in ayurveda medicine in India. Do they really profess ayurveda? Are they scientists in its true meaning? How do they look at science? Is ayurveda a scientific medicine? Can scientific medicine and ayurveda coexist? I answer these questions after outlining the history of ayurveda.

The transliteration scheme helps to understand the pronunciation of Sanskrit words used in this book.

Potturu Ranganayakulu

Foreword

Traditional Medicines are always considered as a nation's pride and many nations and tribes extol their traditions. Acupuncture and moxa in China, kampo in Japan, ayurveda in India, variants of ayurveda in Srilanka, Tibet, Burma; Greek and Arabic traditions in the Middle East and several folk medical practices in Africa and the rest of the continents stand as examples of legacies of the world's medical past. After India's independence in 1947, it was appropriate to patronize the traditional system of medicine to keep up the promises made during the struggle for independence. Therefore, India has adopted a parallel model, patronizing both western/modern and indigenous systems of medicine to address the health needs of India. Now, India has become the second most populous country after China and therefore, an integral part of the growing world economy. The presence of large Indian diasporas the world over has created a big market for Indian traditional medicine. As a result, ayurveda has been gaining currency across the world as one of the preferred alternative systems of medicine.

The growth of scientific medicine cannot entirely replace traditional medicine. The ideas contributed by traditional systems of medicine can have a greater say in day-to-day health matters. People seek information on diet supplements, herbs, dos and don'ts etc. The World Health Organization looks at the traditional systems of medicine for its practical value in protecting the health of the individual. WHO plans ‘policy’, expects ‘safety’, ‘efficacy’, ‘quality’ and ‘accessibility’ to people and aims at rational use of the traditional systems of medicine. Proper understanding of the history of each system of medicine is useful to plan content and delivery mechanisms of health care industry.

The history of medicine is a story of human experience with health and disease through the ages. Historians of medicine explore every aspect of growth and expansion of traditional systems of medicine as well as the evolution of scientific medicine. Reconstruction of an authentic history of ayurveda is one of the important issues in the history of medicine.

Ayurveda is conventional, time-honored traditional Indian system of medicine native to the subcontinent. In Sanskrit language *āyu* means ‘life’ and/or ‘long life’; *veda* means ‘knowledge’. Ayurveda (the knowledge of long life or energetic life) is an integral part of the Indian heritage and a living tradition as well. Ayurveda is viewed as one of the disciplines of *Indian* science and technology. Ayurveda hospitals have been attracting millions of patients every day. However, the number of studies on the history of ayurveda is relatively fewer than studies on other traditional disciplines like music, architecture, sculpture and philosophy of India. Ayurveda has to redefine its role in India's health-care industry because the modern medicine, popularly known as English medicine, has dominated the Indian medical establishment.

Ayurveda, being a mosaic of folk and tribal healing practices, captured the beliefs of people living and migrated into the Indian subcontinent during the last few thousand years. The approach to understand health and longevity, disease and death in the pre- and proto historic Indian subcontinent underwent a sea change with the entry of new tribes with new perspectives and experiences. A wave of urbanization and Sanskritization during the last 3000 years has helped to fuse the pluralistic medical beliefs and practices into an apparently *complete* medical system, ayurveda, which survived the Islamic and English periods.

Origin and Evolution of Ayurveda

Major religions in India each have their own claims on the origin of medicine and medical science from their Gods. Medical alchemists in India believe in Śiva as the lord of medicine. According to the tradition of Jainism all knowledge was revealed to Jain sages by 'the protector'. *Prāṇavāya* (medicine) is one of the twelve divisions of this revealed knowledge. The*Siddha* school of medicine owes its existence to the sage Agastya.

The important treatises of ayurveda, the *Carakasamhita* and the *Suśrutasamhita* claim the origins of ayurveda to be the creator Brahma, who revealed this knowledge to Indra. The duo Aśvini gods have learned ayurveda from Indra and transmitted it to Ātreya, who had six students. Among the students of Ātreya, Agniveśa and Bhela are well known, because their treatises are available today. The *Agniveśasamhita* is now known as the

Carakasamhita. A major portion of the *Bhelasamhita* is also available now. The *Carakasamhita* mostly deals with internal medicine (treating diseases with medicines). The School of Surgery has another proponent, Dhanvantari, the king of Kāśi. Suśruta was the student of Dhanvantari, who later compiled the *Suśrutasamhita*.

All treatises of ayurveda unanimously propagate the idea that the knowledge of ayurveda is divine, complete and finite. It is viewed as pristine and ageless. However, in the history of ayurveda six phases can be reckoned: the prehistoric period, the Vedic period, the classical period, the medieval period, the colonial phase and the 'new age'. The principles of ayurveda were not created in one place at one time; instead, they show a steady progression through different epochs. Many of the basic principles of ayurveda do not have any practical value because techniques of therapy precede theories of drug action. In traditional systems of medicine, therapeutic practices are older than concepts that appear to explain the way medicines work.

The Prehistoric period of Indian history ends after the fall of the Indus Valley civilization. There is evidence to conclude that the people of the Indus Valley civilization had a good sense of hygiene. The common bathhouses, drainage systems etc. found in the excavated sites of this civilization substantiate these claims. Treatment in this period was mostly related to shamanism and exorcism. Until the Indus script is deciphered satisfactorily, the wealth of information about the state of medicine and physicians in the Indus Valley is difficult to understand. Public sanitation and personal hygiene play a crucial role in preventive medicine and this occupied a prominent place in the Harappa culture. The pictures on the Indus seals suggest that physicians used magic and herbs to treat the majority of diseases. Animism was also in practice. Surgery might be in a preliminary stage, limited only to the extent of lancing boils and immobilizing fractured bones. The contemporary river valley civilizations, Egyptian and Sumerian, have certainly exchanged understanding in medicine with the 'meluha' or Indus civilization. The Indus river valley was just 2000 km away from the inter-reverine civilization between the Euphrates and Tigris in Iraq. The sea route from Indus to Sumeria is shorter than the distance from the Indus to the southern tip of India.

Several tribes, contemporary with the Indus civilization, inhabiting the Indian subcontinent were already using some valuable herbs to treat diseases, which later entered the pharmacopeia of ayurveda. The tribes which migrated to the Malabar (Kerala) region of India thousands of years ago, have discovered several spice yielding plants like pepper, long pepper, cinnamon etc. for their medicinal value in food and medicine. These spices later influenced not only ayurveda but also the history of the world. The tribes of northern India have discovered certain important grains like rice, herbs like turmeric and tamarind and started using them in cuisine and medicine. Undeniably, the roots of ayurveda were pre-Aryan.

The word *ayurveda* is not found in the Vedic literature. It is certainly post-Vedic in origin. The four *Vedas* viz. *Ṛgveda, Yajurveda, Sāmaveda* and *Atharvaveda* carry several references and descriptions of the art and science of healing. The *Atharvaveda*, being the latest, carries more information on medicine. There are several quotations in the *Atharvaveda* prescribing medicinal plants, chants, prayers and appeals to gods employed in healing ailments. Hence, ayurveda is referred to as an affiliate of *Atharvaveda*. The nature of the medicine in the Vedic period was magico-religious in nature. However, the medical knowledge of *Atharvaveda* is not entirely magico-religious; part of it is empirico-rational. The Vedic people prayed to several trees with 'special powers' to heal and these plants later gained entry into the ayurveda pharmacopoeia. The power of prayers in healing was given due emphasis in ayurveda. The Vedic age ended roughly around the 8th century B.C. The classical age or the 'age of treatises' followed the Vedic age.

The age of treatises, from about the 8th century B.C. until the 8th century AD, was dominated by Jainism and Buddhism. These two religions have given form and shape to the medical knowledge of ancient India. During this period, an unknown sage used the term *ayurveda* to indicate the knowledge of medicine. The monks of the Jainism and Buddhism collated and compiled the people's expertise of medicine and thus, ayurveda evolved as an independent medical discipline. When the Jain and Buddhist monks traveled across the Indian subcontinent to preach, they were exposed to several healing practices in vogue among the people. Several authors have composed *samhitas*, the medical encyclopedias. This period provided three masterpieces of ayurveda, which are popularly known as The Great Three (*bṛhatrayi*): the *Carakasamhita,* the*Suśrutasamhita*and the *Aṣṭāngahṛdaya*. There were scores of other treatises but content-wise they were similar.

The word *samhita* means collection or compilation. The know-how of the laity, born out of experience with Mother Nature, was later codified by scholars in the form of *samhitas*. Later, when Jainism and Buddhism declined, the treatises of ayurveda yielded to the influence of Brahmanism in philosophical outlook.

These medical treatises describe every aspect of life with emphasis on how to stay healthy. The main objective of the *samhita* is to help preserve health and achieve emancipation from rebirth. The daily regimen, seasonal regimen, good conduct, augury, prayers are prescribed to avoid diseases. Hundreds of plants and several animal products like milk, ghee, gallstones, urine, and horns were used to formulate medicines. Ayurveda became enriched with folklore therapies from the four corners of India. A quote from *Ṛgveda* says 'let noble thoughts flow from all directions'. The spirit of the Vedic people has helped ayurveda to imbibe the best of India's medical heritage.

Medieval Period

It is commonly held by historians of medicine that in the medieval period, from the Islamic invasions in 10th c. AD until the dissolution of the Mughal Empire in the 18th c. AD, ayurveda was eclipsed by political and cultural hostilities. In spite of the weakening state patronage, ayurveda scholars produced quite a number of treatises, dictionaries/thesauri (*Nighaṇṭu*), commentaries and translations. The Lesser Triad (*laghutrayi*), comprising the *Mādhavanidāna*, the *Bhāvaprakāśa* and the *Śārangadhara*, were composed during this period.

The medieval period has provided many sources of epigraphy referring to ayurveda. The social status of ayurveda physicians continued to be very high, but it started experiencing a downturn. In some kingdoms, some physicians received corporal punishments for their failures. Vigorous trade relations with the West initiated some changes. New plants and food items were introduced into India. New medicinal formulations were invented, and new diseases spread from other parts of the world into India.

Alchemy was and is one of the secret sciences of India, across the entire length and breadth of the country. Many Ayurveda physicians have pursued the art of making gold out of mercury! The search for miracle cures was intensified. The universities that once flourished in Nalanda, Taxila, Ujjain, Kasi and other places had gradually declined. Ayurvedic education at a university standard that had flourished once during the Buddhist period disappeared. Many Indians believe the universities in ancient India were similar to the universities now. However, the ancient Indian universities focused on religious studies and languages. In spite of their existence for more than 800 years, modern linguistics and natural sciences had not evolved. India had to wait for modern science from European universities during the colonial age. Academic freedom is the soul of the universities.

The hostile political environment, orthodoxy, aloofness, distance and lack of communications between the isolated scholars were prime factors for diminished productivity and lack of creativity in general science and medicine. Against all these odds, the medieval period did produce more compositions and invented equally more medicinal formulations. However, these inventions and discoveries did not pave the way to scientific medicine. An important feature of ayurvedic education in the medieval period is the disappearance of universities and institutionalized education. Ayurveda continued in the hermitage system.

The medieval period is very important in the history of ayurveda. Because it was during this period, that the changes that took place in Siddha medicine influenced ayurveda in the south. The examination of *nāḍi* (pulse) of *aṣṭasthānaparīkṣa* (eightfold examination) became important techniques in the diagnostics of ayurveda. The regional variations of ayurveda were clearer than earlier. In this age, yunani, Islamic medicine, joined the stream and rivaled ayurveda. The popularity of yunani medicine however did not diminish the chances of ayurveda. Although pharmaceutical products increased in number during the medieval period, conceptual growth had struck a dead-end because of religious orthodoxy and unwillingness to learn new things.

The Colonial Period

The fall of the Vijayangara Empire in the 16th century AD and subsequent developments in polity and politics, like the fragile Mughal Empire and the maritime adventures of Europeans, led to the British filling the power-vacuum in the Indian subcontinent. British trade and the new Indian economy drastically altered the nature of medicine. Burgeoning European medicine touched the shores of India and made a big dent on ayurveda. More than the European medicine, the inventions and discoveries in science and technology and the new British administration greatly altered the shape of ayurveda. Several British and continental European travelers travelled across India and recorded their observations on the principles and practice of ayurveda. Their chronicles are highly useful to understand the status of ayurveda in medieval India. The British established the first Government College in Calcutta in 1822 to train the native doctors to serve the British army. The British Orientalists, who supported Indian culture and the Anglicists, who wanted to *modernize* India by English education, disputed over the nature of ayurvedic education. The greatest contribution of the colonial rule to ayurveda was the accessibility to printing technology. Many ayurveda treatises were printed on paper for the first time. This was a real democratic process triggering integration of ayurveda with other systems of medicine. The process of secularization of ayruveda was initiated.

The renaissance of ayurveda started in Bengal and gradually started spreading to other parts of India. Ayurveda physicians were divided into two ideological camps, one group aspiring for purity in ayurveda teaching and practice, and the other seeking integration of ayurveda with the emerging western medicine. The British administration had established a series of committees to solve the problems of medical education, but when the British had to leave India in 1947, they bequeathed the problems of ayurveda administration to the new Indian Government.

New Age Ayurveda

Mahatma Gandhi disapproved of the obsolete ideology of ayurveda physicians. Though Gandhi applied Naturopathy for himself and his family, he did not support integrated medicine. The so-called visionaries of India in the 19th and 20th centuries could not visualize a feasible system of medicine for independent India. After India's independence, for practical reasons, the Government of India encouraged modern medicine. Though the Government of India supported ayurvedic education, ayurveda physicians did not plan their future in independent India. In the 1960s and 70s, many intellectuals felt that the

Complementary and Alternative Medicines (CAM) were losing ground, but, those supporting CAM systems did find some new ground to stand on. The religious gurus from India were exploiting ayurveda just to earn fame and fortune abroad. The (mis)interpretations of the concepts of ayurveda by some Hindu gurus and a few cosmopolitan ayurveda physicians have given a new lease of life to ayurveda. Feeding on the ignorance of the people has become a lifestyle for many cosmopolitan ayurveda physicians and 'religious gurus'. In India, you can still find ayurveda physicians, qualified or unqualified, giving medicine to help conceive a male baby, to treat juvenile diabetes, cancers, HIV so on and so forth.

The new age ayurveda is marked by several syncretic writings. Syncretic means trying to reconcile, often unsuccessfully, differing schools of thought in convincing rationality. Syncretism has entered into every aspect of ayurveda, such as anatomy and physiology, pathology and medicine. Several writings by both Indian and Western ayurveda scholars try to claim that ayurveda constitutes a revolution in what they claim is an ideal system of medicine. Ayurveda medicines are claimed to be without any undesirable effects. People believe in these new claims. However, vestiges of religion and belief abound in the theory and practice of ayurveda.

The advent of the internet has hastened the process of commercialization of ayurveda the world over. Popular writers use smart language to write about ayurveda. Attractive WebPages hide absurd and outdated concepts. Ayurvedic medicines are marketed in alluring packs. Hundreds of international conferences and seminars happen in India and abroad. Ayurvedic tourism has added Kerala as one of the top twenty tourist destinations in the world. All this pomp is New Age Ayurveda.

Ayurveda claims the title of 'complete' medicine because it has its own versions of anatomy, physiology, pathology and medicine. Can science measure this totality of ayurveda? The government of India recognizes ayurveda as an independent and complete medical system. This attitude has become a major obstacle in the development of a comprehensive medical care in India.

Chapter One
DRAVIDIAN ROOTS OF AYURVEDA

When a lot of remedies are suggested for a disease that means it cannot be cured.

– Anton Chekhov (1860 – 1904)

A traditional system of medicine is a product of human experience with disease and death. According to the World Health Organization, traditional medicine is 'the sum total of knowledge, skills and practices based on theories, beliefs and experiences indigenous to different cultures that are put in use to maintain health, and prevent, diagnose, improve or treat physical as well as mental illnesses.' There are hundreds of traditional medical systems indigenous to different biological and cultural milieu and these medical traditions are in constant slow flux. Ethno-medicine and ethno-biology study the interrelations between several systems of medicine and human experience with plants and animals. All dominant traditional medical systems tend to be on collision courses or amalgamations with one another. When a civilization thrives, its system of medicine naturally blooms and reaches places beyond its original borders, leading to exchanges between civilizations. Raw material for medicines like mercury, herbs etc. figured prominently in the list of international merchandise since prehistoric times. Egyptian, Sumerian, Indus and Chinese civilizations were in contact with one another. Ancient civilizations in Greece, India and China promoted exchange of scholars and ambassadors. All schools of medicine learned from one another and so no system of medicine can claim to be a virgin.

Compared with the Himalayas on a geological timescale, ayurveda is a recent cultural phenomenon of the Indian subcontinent. The development of ayurveda owes much to the rich experience of several ethnic groups living in the Indian subcontinent for several thousands of years. Ayurveda is seen as Aryan medicine or Hindu medicine. However, there is no such entity, unlike Dravidian medicine. The word dravida is used to refer to the heritage of south India. There is a Dravidian language family and Dravidian culture in contrast to that of Aryan culture and languages. Historians of medicine have not paid sufficient attention to the contributions of Dravidian culture to Hindu medicine. Now, Siddha medicine occupies the place previously called Dravidian medicine.

It is unclear how the word Dravida formed. Some feel it is a derivation of the word *dramila* in the Buddhist literature referring to the southern province. South India is the bastion of Dravidian culture. Before the arrival of Aryan tribes into the Indian subcontinent, the dominant and numerous Dravidian and Austric tribes, speaking several Dravidian and Austric languages populated many habitable regions of the entire subcontinent. The Negritos (out of Africa) were the first settlers in the Indian subcontinent, and they were followed by the Austric and Dravidian tribes. Austric people entered India from the east, mostly from Southeast Asia. By the time of the Aryan spread, Dravidians had absorbed several cultural elements from earlier tribes. Dravidians were the first to leave the marks of their culture on literature and architecture of India. Due to the gradual spread of the Aryan tribes from the north, Dravidians were slowly pushed to the east and peninsular south. Earlier, the description of *Draviḍadeśa* was equated to the entire Indian subcontinent, but now it represents only South India, where Dravidian languages, including Tamil, Telugu, Kannada and Malayalam are spoken by more than 250 million people.

The People of India

A hallmark of India is its racial and linguistic diversity. Modern times have given the subcontinent its nationality and India has never been as big as it is today. During the last few millennia, many different racial groups converged into India leading to the emergence of one of the most ancient societies of the world. For example, great population movements were recorded during the 6th and 7th centuries AD. Great migrations took place during the Indus civilization and continued until the 20th century. However, Around 1000 AD, the population ratios of various tribes and castes in India had become stabilized.

The Negritos comprised the oldest group of people to enter India. They did not know how to make instruments and so there was neither agriculture nor housing. *Erukala*, *Kurumba* in south India and Onge in the Andamans islands are a few examples of this group of people. The Austric (proto-Australoid) group of people followed Negritos. Tribes linked to the Austric are found in central and southeast India. The Munda and Santhal tribes of eastern India belong to this category. They are known as *āgneya* (southeast) people. Mongoloid tribes (Tibeto-Burman) people entered the subcontinent from the northeast and Tibet region; the *Māram* tribe of Manipur belongs to this group. The Proto-Dravidians are Mediterranean in origin and reached the subcontinent by land and sea; the *Gonds* of central India provide an example of this group. Later, some Dravidian groups became more urbanized. The Indus civilization is assumed to be the product of Dravidians. The Nordics or Aryans is the most important group of people migrating into India. Many Aryan tribes from the central Asian region continued to replace the urban culture of the Indus river valley in the second millennium BC. Most of the Brahmins and tribes like gypsies and *sugalis* belong to Aryan group.

The phrases 'scheduled tribes', 'scheduled castes' and 'backward classes' are relatively new and revised categories to describe the people of India. During the colonial rule, British anthropologists and sociologists, especially Edgar Thurston and others, have studied the people of India and documented the traits of all tribes and castes. Caste and tribe are two crucial words that dominate the Indian psyche. The word tribe is used for a group of people still adhering to their traditional lifestyle, hunting, shifting cultivation etc. and residing in their traditional habitat. The schedule tribe category described by the Government of India includes several groups of tribes that belong to any of the Negrito, Aryan, Dravidian or Tibetan groups still cherishing their traditional way of life. A group of people labelled ‘scheduled tribe’ by the Government of India deserves special support in education and employment. All these tribes are economically and socially backward, and remain under-privileged, away from the mainstream.

The percentage of tribal populations in different parts of India gives us some clues for understanding the demography of India. The extent to which a region's population is tribal varies considerably from north to south. In the northeastern states of Arunachal Pradesh, Meghalaya, Mizoram, and Nagaland, over ninety percent of the population is tribal. In the remaining northeast states of Assam, Manipur, Sikkim, and Tripura it is between twenty and thirty percent of the total population. The largest tribes are found in central India, although the tribal population accounts for only around ten percent of the region's total population. In the south, just one percent of the population of Kerala and Tamil Nadu are tribal, whereas six percent of the population of Andhra Pradesh and Karnataka are of tribal stock. This variation proves that the tribes were migrating from north to the south slowly. Therefore, the majority of the present south Indian population has migrated more rapidly than the tribes during the last two millennia. More migrations took place during the Jain and Buddhist periods, bringing in Aryan elements into language and social life. Some tribes have taken the maritime route to reach India. Thiyya and Ezhava tribes are known for their association with medicinal herbs in Kerala from time immemorial. The Thiyya tribe left Kyrgyzstan and reached Kerala seven thousand years ago. The Ezhavas migrated to south India from Srilanka.

Today, the five hundred and thirty tribes of India comprise around seventy million people. They mainly subsist on fishing and produce from the forests. In spite of several welfare measures, most of the indigenous population of India is still out of the mainstream. Some groups of people, derived from several tribes, have left mountainous regions and occupied cultivable plain lands as farmers and artisans. They distanced from their tribes and their proportion of the population has increased over and above the tribal population. The division of labor divided the people into castes but it lubricated the economy.

Caste poses a big problem to sociologists. Historically caste groups emerged from different races or several tribes at different periods. Populations, who discarded their tribal identity, took to caste, each caste being an endogamous group involved in a specific economic activity. 'Scheduled castes' are at the periphery of Hindu society, participating in the economy by fulfilling unclean but essential services. The backward caste category includes hundreds of groups of people like agriculturists, artisans and other professionals belonging to livestock and diary. All castes arising from Aryan tribes do not necessarily belong to the upper strata and some caste groups arising from Negrito, Austric and Dravidians belong to dominant caste groups. Thus, the caste is a new form of tribe.

It was possible for the so-called lower caste people to experience upward movement. Many kingdoms and empires in India were built by the underprivileged sections. When political power gave them any advantage, they were hinduized by the priest class. The Vijayanagara Empire (14th C.) was founded by Harihara and Bukka, who belonged to the shepherd caste. When certain underprivileged groups of people attain political power, their family history is rewritten lauding their heroic adventures. Therefore, the caste is a 'cultured' form of tribe. Oral histories of several castes also attest and concur with this transformation.

Ways of cremation too reveal racial differences in India. More castes in south India dispose of the dead by burial. The Aryan way of disposal is by cremation. The Dravidian practice is dominant in south India. Fire-worship is most popular among the population groups that migrated into India from the Middle East.

Recent studies in genetics give irrefutable evidence for the migration patterns of different population groups. In an article titled *Genetic evidence on the origins of Indian caste populations*, eighteen scholars, mainly from Utah in the US and Andhra University in Andhra Pradesh, India, led by Michael Bamshad of the Department of Pediatrics from the University of Utah make the claim that there were several waves of immigration into India, the last of which (from Europe) was solely responsible for the caste system. It says, the Indo-European speaking people from West Eurasia entered India from the Northwest and diffused throughout the subcontinent. They purportedly admixed with or displaced Dravidic-speaking populations. Subsequently, they may have established caste system and probably placed themselves in castes of higher rank. The Genographic study undertaken by the National Geographic Society emphasizes a similar pattern. The results of such studies will have political and cultural ramifications for India.

Pre-Aryan Tribes and Proto-Medicine

Disease and death are natural to all species of life and healing techniques are as old as human evolution. Surprisingly some of them were learnt from apes and other animals. The historians of medicine understand these developments clearly, if they happened in the recent past but our understanding of developments in medical history gets blurred, as we go back in time. Studies of medicine in the Old and New Stone Ages are based not on documentary evidence but on archaeological excavations and conjecture.

Evolution of humans started long after continental drift had broken the super continent Pangea into the present pattern of a global mosaic of continents. At the end of the Cretaceous period (c. 145 – 66 million years ago), India was still far away from Asia and the Himalayan mountain range was non-existent. Hominids evolved in the Pleistocene age (2.58 million years to 11,700 years ago). Although some hominids (Ramapithecus) were populating the plains of northern India, it was African species of Homo sapiens that spread into the Indian subcontinent. Ramapithecus is not considered as fully human by the anthropologists. According to the theory of 'Out of Africa', human migration along the coast towards the east first brought humans into the Indian subcontinent. These people, Negritos, stepped into India at least 50,000 years ago. Progress in human civilization was slow but steady. Humans used stone projectiles as weapons at least 1.8 million years ago and fire was used with caution at least a million years ago. These changes led to other milestones in the journey to progress. At least500,000 years ago purpose-built shelters were erected. 100,000 years ago ostrich egg shells were used to transport water. At the same time shell jewelry and ochre body paints were used. 70,000 years ago, humans started wearing clothes and the oldest needle dates back to 60,000 years ago. The earliest ritualistic burial dated back to 50,000 years ago and the oldest cave artists 35,000 years old. The plough was invented 8000 years ago and the first writing occurred 5000 years ago. Amid these milestones of human civilization, the use of herbs as medicines too spans back thousands of years. A pottery cauldron containing boiled medicinal herbs unearthed in 2001 in Zhejiang Province of China indicates that Neolithic people used natural herbal medicine as early as 8,000 years ago. These inventions and discoveries spread to other cultures slowly.

Neolithic technologies, originated in the Middle East around 9000 BC, spread eastward to the Indus river valley by 5000 BC where man started farming, using metal, bricks and pottery. Farming communities based on millet and rice appeared in the Huang Ho (Yellow River) valley of China and in Southeast Asia by about 3500 BC. Neolithic modes of life developed independently in the new world (Americas). Corn (maize), beans, and squash were gradually domesticated in Mexico and Central America from 6500 BC onwards, though sedentary village life did not commence there until much later, at about 2000 BC. In the old world (Asia, Africa and Europe) the Neolithic period was succeeded by the bronze age, when human societies learned to combine copper and tin to make bronze, which replaced stone for use as tools and weapons. The proximity of the Indus river valley to the 'fertile crescent' in the Middle East helped exchanges in the field of food production since prehistoric times and the alphabetization of language was a result of leisure in the river valley civilizations.

Scalpels made of obsidian, a naturally occurring volcanic 'glass', by the upper Paleolithic blade techniques were discovered in archaeological excavations. Some operations were done using these scalpels by modern surgeons and proved effective because these scalpels made from natural material are very efficient. The Neolithic period started about 12,000 years ago, this phase was marked by domestication of animals and plants. Goats, which habituated to hilly terrain, were brought to the plains by the people in the Fertile Crescent. Sheep were kept at ancient Jericho 9000 years ago. Several animals and birds were first domesticated in the Indian subcontinent. *Punjiṣṭa*, an Indian tribe, derived its name from their pioneering discovery and domestication of fowl. A tribe *Svanin* domesticated wild dogs. A Munda group known as *niṣāda* first discovered turmeric in nature and started using it in food and medicine.

They domesticated birds, animals and plants, which helped reduce the hard work of hunting and made life easier. Domestication also helped to breed plants and animals in many ways. Such plants need not 'struggle' for existence, so the edible parts, like fruits, tubers, seeds etc. could grow in size and flavor.

Civilizations in different parts of the world discovered metals, wheels and fire. Unleavened bread is a late Neolithic discovery. At that time, 5000 years ago, the population of the world was just 10 million. Gradually the population of India grew, because of the fertility of the soil and timely monsoons. Demographers guess that the population of India became 10 million 2000 years ago. The Indus civilization, which was contemporary with the civilizations in China, Middle East and Egypt, made steady progress on several fronts in medicine, but we are unable to understand its contributions, because the script has not yet been deciphered. However, it is presumed that treatment in the Indus culture mostly involved magic and sorcery. Approximately 5000 seals from the Indus valley and the Middle East have been recovered, but they are unintelligible to researchers. Several hypotheses have been tested using frontline technology to decipher the script. Ayurveda and its theories were probably unknown to the Indus people. However, the use of salts, acquired from mountains, riverbeds and quarries, as medicine might have been in vogue among the Indus people.

Shared common ancestry and similarities in human psychology are the prime cause of resemblances in beliefs in medical systems in all human societies. Humans conjectured the existence of supernatural forces or gods and regarded disease and death as results of a curse or of past actions. Treatments were discovered in nature, animals contributing a great deal to evidence-based medical treatment. Humans observed animals and learned some properties of herbs. Inventions and discoveries were mostly accidental at that time. In surgery too, ancient men achieved some progress. Remains of human settlements in the lower, middle and upper Paleolithic and Mesolithic periods have been unearthed in different parts of India. Megaliths, Neolithic settlements, are found in almost all parts of south India. People call them *pānḍavagullu* (habitations of Pandava) or *rakasigullu* (habitations of giants). Several megalithic sites have yielded iron implements like horse stirrups, ladles, arrowheads and vessels. Surgery was in its primitive phase at this time and was perhaps limited to eliciting broken thorns from the soles and puncturing wounds filled with pus. Surgical utensils were probably limited to extracting arrowheads from the bodies of animals and humans. However, the hard metal, iron, hastened the progress of agriculture and surgery. Many of the urban habitations established in the early part of first millennium B.C. had grown into centers of trade and culture in the *Śātavāhana* period by the later part of the first millennium B.C.

Many excavated sites show urban occupations lasting up to around the 3rd century AD. Archaeological excavations have yielded information about the food habits and health traditions of these people. Plant remains that have been identified include kodo millet (Paspalum scrobiculatum), barley (hordeum vulgare), hyacinth bean (dolichos lablab), horse gram (dolichos biflors), black gram (vigna mungo), common pea (pisum arvense) and rice (oryza sativa). Vegetarian diets during the Megalithic phase were supplemented by wild game, birds and aquatic fauna. The remains of black buck (antelope cervicapra), sambar (cervus unicolor), chital (axis axis), hare (lepus nigricollis), porcupine (hystrix indica), fowls, tortoises and mollusc's shells have been unearthed.

Early Medicine in India

Medicine is as old as humankind is. Human societies across the world have reacted to disease and death spontaneously. At times of sickness, they have searched for remedies in nature and knowledge of these remedies was exchanged between cultures. However, the sickness is unrelenting and the desire to escape from sickness eventually ushered in the way to scientific medicine. The efforts of Indian culture related to the growth of scientific medicine are discussed in the ensuing pages.

A good place to understand the lifestyle of the early Indians is at Bhimbetka in Madhya Pradesh where there are more than 600 natural caves used by the primitive man as home. Only 12 caves are now open for visitors. The paintings in these caves date from the prehistoric to the medieval age, the oldest painting going back to 12000 B.C. and the most recent to 1000 AD. Some paintings in these caves show the animal giraffe and the ostrich bird. K.T. Achaya in his 'History of Indian Food' opines that these animals might have been hunted to extinction. This may not be a fact because human habitations in the past were relatively less dense to enable them to become extinct by hunting and a pestilence or disease might have wiped out certain species of animals.

During this period of activity around Bhimbetka, several groups of people living in different eco-climatic zones befriended the surrounding nature. Apparently, four important streams of population movement have participated in the growth of medicine in India. The Negrito, first settlers in India, did not know how to make instruments. They did not even have agriculture or housing. Anthropologists have discovered that the Negrito people worshiped the 'banyan' tree and identified tens of plants useful in food and medicine. The proto-australoid or austric people are mostly found in the central and southeast India; the *Santhal, Munda, Birhor, Asur, Korba, Coorg, Juang* tribes belong to this group. They had pickaxes and primitive agriculture, growing rice, banana, brinjals, lemon, jamboo fruit, cotton and coconut. Herbal medicine must have taken root in this period, because the use of several useful herbs like coconut, lime, rice etc. play an important role in Indian medicine. These people believed in rebirth, incarnation of a god as a tortoise and pantheism; that is every natural being is godly. Therefore, rivers, mountains, sky, celestial objects etc are seen as the forms of god. They had stories about the origin and creation of the universe. They could distinguish between the eatables and non-eatables.

This distinction can be achieved only after sustained experimentation with nature. Their accumulated knowledge was transmitted to the other cultures of India. Several elements of Hinduism have roots in these beliefs and practices of the Austric people of India. The ayurvedic concept of *ātma* (soul) dates to this era.

Dravidians discovered sandal, and practiced incense burning and prayer (*puja*). They worshiped Hanuman, Siva, Uma, Kartikeya. The Indus civilization abruptly halted in the second millennium B.C. The Aryan migration during the Indus civilization has altered the course of Indian history forever. A group of new Aryan languages started absorbing the elements of ancient Indian culture, which was Dravidian or pre-Dravidian.

Anthropologists have documented the medical beliefs and practices of almost all the tribes of India. Tribal medicine too was not frozen in time and over a period; the contents of tribal medicine underwent several changes. Each tribe would have a sorcerer, soothsayer, magician and an herb-healer. Although there is no specific entity that can be labeled Dravidian medicine, the diversified practices of ancient tribes of India can be summed up as Dravidian medicine. Ayurveda had borrowed heavily from these tribes. Tamarind, coconut, pigeon pea (Cajanus cajan), betel leaf and many herbs were discovered in south India for their medicinal values.

K.T. Achaya gives an interesting history of ayurvedic herbs in *The Story of Our Food*. Old words of several herbs, fruits etc from the Munda language have entered the Sanskrit vocabulary: *Nimbuka* for neem, *Injavera* for ginger, *chinchāphala* for tamarind, *guvaka* for betel nut, *vrintaka* for brinjal, *panasa* for jackfruit all come from non-Aryan languages of India and enriched the Sanskrit. The most important of all is rice, the staple food in south India. The Sanskrit word for rice is *vrihi* or *varisi*. The Tamil word *arisi* is the mother of these words. It even entered into English as rice. The Hindi word *chaval* for rice also come from another Munda word *chom-la*. Rice was first domesticated and cultivated near water bodies in north India by the pre-Aryan tribes.

The English word curry too comes from Tamil *kari*, which means a dish cooked with pepper. Pepper is native to south India. Mango is *āmra* in Sanskrit. The Tamil word *mānga* is the mother of all words related to mango. Mango is native to the Indian subcontinent so the pre-Aryan tribes identified its value in food. Therefore, the roots of ayurveda spring from Dravidian and pre-dravidian lifestyles. Pigeon-pea (Cajanus cajan), black gram (Vigna mungo), green gram (Vigna radiata), horse gram (Macrotyloma uniflorum)were discovered in the Indian subcontinent. The chickpea comes from Turkey-Syria and the lentil (masur) comes from southwest Asia (Turkey-Cyprus). The diversity of edible plant species in the subcontinent made the people living in India to esteem vegetarian diet. D.D. Kosambi, a pioneer in the history of India, says 'food gathering apart from hunting or fishing remained much easier over most of India and had a far greater range than in Europe or elsewhere on the Eurasian continent. Where half a dozen cereals, peas and beans make up almost the entire variety of European staple foods, even a region of average fertility like Maharashtra has over 40 kinds of indigenous vegetarian staples, most of which are cultivated but can also be found wild. All are suitable for storing. These include rice and wheat, millets, sorghum, barley; with a considerable variety of vegetable proteins, and seeds like sesame that produce edible oil. Pepper and spices provide good flavor and serve as medicinal plants as well. A balanced diet was possible without killing any living creatures. Milk, butter, curds and cheese are available without sacrificing animal life. This simple fact was later to revolutionize Indian theology and religion with the doctrine of non-killing (ahimsa).

Before the advent of Aryan medical knowledge in India, the folk therapies of the tribes were heterogeneous and decentralized, there being no cultural or political force to bring uniformity in the practice of medicine. Medical service was a pastime apart from the main occupation and was mostly hereditary. Ordinary language was used to talk to the patient. Occult treatment and animism were popular and these practices are still seen in India. The sick were placed near the confluence of rivers or streams for recovery. They prayed to banana plants, when women could not be impregnated. Pestilence and epidemics were considered as curse by supernatural forces. In spite of new cultures and technologies entering India, old practices in medicine continue to thrive, because the tribes are mainly endogamous, and India is often therefore referred to as an ethnological museum by indologists. Therefore, the kind of medicine that was prevalent in pre-Aryan India is still being practiced in several parts of India. The Anthropological Survey of India (ASI) has documented the medical practices of several tribes of India and the records show close resemblances in customs and beliefs in medicine among different tribes living over great distances from one another.

The *Savara* tribe in Orissa and Andhra Pradesh believed in the curse of gods as the causative factor of diseases like blindness, cough, insanity, eclampsia (a toxic condition of pregnancy) and they believed in appeasing gods. All tribes believed in some physical causes of diseases, including eating non-edibles and bad weather. Relief is sought from *janni*, a priest, *ejjodu*, a shaman, who identifies the reasons and prescribes treatments to the *Savara* and *Jatapu* tribes. The healers have different names like *dissari, guravadu, vejju, vejjuralu. Vejju* is similar to the Pali and Sanskrit terms for doctor, *vaidya*.

The*Chenchu* tribe on the banks of the river Krishna use different herbs and animal products in treating diseases and every member of the Chenchu tribe is *vaidya*! The *Chenchus* roam south India with their medical kits. They appear in market towns and roadsides offering incredible treatments for everything from fevers to snakebites. They use turmeric with burned and ground legs of peacock for the common cold; *Nelavemu* (Andrographis paniculata) for fevers; seeds of the silk cotton tree (Butea monosperma) for intestinal worms; cauterization of the wrist for jaundice; the leaves of *tulsi* (Ocimum sanctum) for coughing. All these treatments suggest a reminiscent flow of knowledge from tribal systems to mainstream ayurveda. Ayurveda treatises too give equal importance to the divine cause of diseases in several conditions like leprosy, tuberculosis, diabetes etc. Many concepts and treatments used by Indian tribes are accepted in ayurveda. While the tribes remained in their habitations, roaming ascetics (Jain, Buddhist and Brahminic) have compiled the best from all tribal practices into mainstream medicine.

Pepper and long pepper have assumed utmost importance in ayurvedic pharmacopeia. Every ayurvedic preparation contains some pepper and long pepper because these are considered *dipana* and *pācana* (they increase appetite and digestion power) and useful in scores of ailments. These two herbs grow wild in the Malabar Coast of South India. The tribes living in Kerala discovered pepper and long pepper in nature, probably at least eight thousand years ago. The *Pancakarma* (five therapeutic procedures) of ayurveda too has regional variations. The so-called Kerala *pancakarma* has certain methods, *pizzichchil, navarakizhi, dhāra* etc. were not invented by the *Ātreya sampradāya* of ayurveda. These techniques date back to pre-Aryan times and have enriched the therapies of ayurveda in modern times. Therefore, the keraliya therapies are Dravidian in origin.

Dravidian Language and Medical Jargon

'Sanskrit is the mother of all languages' is a popular belief in India. This belief is weakened by discoveries in modern linguistics. Alexander Campbell first proposed the Dravidian language family in 1816 after observing the structures of the Indian languages. However, Robert Caldwell first used the term 'Dravidian' in his book Dravida Grammar. Telugu, Kannada, Tamil and Malayalam are major languages in the Dravidian language family, which is distinct from the Indo-Aryan languages including Sanskrit. The Dravidian languages have contributed countless words to Sanskrit and ayurveda. Words for most of the diseases, signs and symptoms of the diseases, medicinal plants and concepts in ayurveda come from the Dravidian and Munda languages. Therefore, the study of the words for diseases contributes to the history of medicine, providing an extra perspective.

The Munda language group belongs to the Austro-Asiatic family of languages (spoken in Southeast Asia), much older than the Dravidian family in the Indian subcontinent. The Austric super family of languages was proposed by Wilhelm Schmidt in 1906. The Santhal language of eastern India belongs to this group. The Munda languages are spoken in Bihar, Jarkhand, Orissa and central India. There was exchange of vocabulary between the Dravidian languages and Munda languages much before the entry of Sanskrit. The Sanskrit language, a late arrival into India, has borrowed medical vocabulary from both of these language groups.

The Dravidian family of languages contains 26 distinct languages. By 1100 B.C. these languages could be placed into three subgroups, southern, central and northern, due to migrations and divergence of the families. The *Brahui* language is an example of the northern group, spoken in Pakistan; Telugu belongs to the south-central group, while Tamil, Malayalam, Kannada and some other languages belong to the southern group.

The Dravidian languages have borrowed more words from the Aryan languages during the last two thousand years, due to the influence of Jain and Buddhist religions. Sanskrit had borrowed structures in grammar; Telugu, for instance, has coexisted with Indo-Aryan languages for more than two thousand years and as a result, the Telugu language has acquired more words from Indo-Aryan languages.

Each noun in Telugu has a pair of words. For instance, 'mother' can be translated to *talli* and *amma*; hill (*konda* and *parvātam*), eye (*kannu* and *akshi*) etc. the first word is Dravidian and the second one is from Sanskrit. The word 'medicine' is *aushadam* and *mandu*. The word *mandu* is Dravidian and *aushadam* is Sanskrit-derived. Therefore, ayurveda carries several Dravidian and proto-Dravidian words used in health science. The Telugu word *mandu* is derived from a proto-Dravidian word *maram,* which indicates a 'tree'. *Mar-untu* is medicine made from herbs. Therefore, *mandu* is a medicinal preparation. We still find the usage of several proto Dravidian words in the medical science of Telugu *viz*.. *netturu* (blood), *potta* (abdomen), *noppi* (pain), *cavu* (death) etc. These words are also found in other Dravidian languages with slight modifications, viz. savu (Kannada), neyttor (Tamil) etc.

The knowledge and wisdom of the aboriginal people of India, stored in their vernacular languages, were slowly extinguished by sanskritization; hence, it is difficult to know the true history of ayurveda and India. Sociologists describe sanskritization as a process of adaptation of non-Aryan tribes to Hindu customs. Sanskritization has absorbed the experience of the people and preserved it in immutable Sanskrit. When the Aryans entered India from the northern temperate regions, they had no words in their vocabulary for a large number of plants, animals and unknown products of the new country, so they acquired important loans from the languages of the Dravidian and pre-Dravidian populations with whom they first came into contact.

The words *Languli, linga* come from the Austro-Asiatic languages and are familiar in the Mon-Khmer languages of south East Asia. They are not found in the Indo-European vocabulary but were borrowed when Sanskrit and other languages entered India. The words *linga* and *lingula* indicates phallus, plough, tail etc. Przyluski and others have elaborately demonstrated the borrowed words from the Austric group of languages to Sanskrit. Study of words and their history is a one of the promising areas that can unlock the true history of ayurveda.

Chapter Two
AYURVEDA IN ANCIENT INDIA

The central doctrine that humoral inequality is identical with disease must be wrong.

-Vireswara in *Rogārogavāda* (1669AD)

The introduction of iron into the Indian subcontinent occurred around 1000 BC. Approximately, at the same period, evidences of use of iron were found in Tungabhadra river valley in south India. Iron implements could improve farm production, give leisure and enhance lifespan. Increase of population necessitates political organization of society. In north India *mahajanapadas* (big clusters of population) originated, which subsequently grew into kingdoms and empires. The empire building and urbanization augmented developments in medicine, literature, art and architecture. The decadent Vedic lifestyle suffered from schisms in the *colored* society. The discrimination and *varṇa*(color) system lead to the rise of Jainism and Buddhism. These two movements originated to quench the thirst of knowledge and deliver justice to the underprivileged sections of the society. Animal sacrifices, privileges to priest class were discouraged. Young students, who were attracted by these new religions, took to asceticism and roamed the subcontinent spreading the word of dharma and compassion. Jainism and Buddhism competed with each other and with the established Brahmanism. The roaming ascetics and mendicants have started collecting and compiling folk therapies into an organized body of medical knowledge.

At this juncture, medical know-how was compiled into *samhitas* (treatises), which were secular in the beginning. Simultaneously, medical information was also recorded in *purāṇas* (scriptures of ancient times), epics and similar non-secular literature. Ayurveda reached its pinnacle between 5th century BC and 5th century AD and for almost one thousand years, it was not challenged by any other school of medicine. Panini and Patanjali systematized the grammar of Sanskrit and saved it from extinction from 4th century BC onwards. Brahmin scholars and Vedic scholars started using revised Sanskrit to communicate with other scholars in far off places surrounded by different vernacular languages like Pali, Magadhi etc. *Agniveśasamhita, Bhelasamhita* and 4 other treatises were authored by 6 disciples of Ātreya at Takshasila, of which only *Bhelasamhita* and *Agniveśasamhita* (in the name of *Carakasamhita*) stood the test of time. However, the knowledge of medicine is partly available in several forms of religious or non-religious compositions. Some Brahmin scholars gave up Vedic learning and dedicated their time to secular sciences like medicine, music and literature.

The knowledge was inherited orally to the ensuing generations in ancient India. The Sanskrit word *bahusṛta* (well educated) literally means 'listened to many'. However, the *devanāgari* and other scripts of India were devised from *Brāhmi* script in northwest India in 4th or 3rd centuries BC. Until these scripts were widely used, ayurveda treatises were part of oral tradition. Historians understood that the *Brāhmi* script was a derived form of Aramaic script of the Middle East. Until now, there are no evidences to prove the genesis of *Brāhmi* script from the pictures of Indus seals. Writing *samhitas* is a recent phenomenon in the history of ayurveda. The oldest copy of the *Carakasamhita* now available belongs to 9th century AD.

Paper is in use in India for about 1000 years. *Kagaj* (paper) and *kitab* (book) are Persian words. Palms (Corypha umbraculifera and Borassus flabelliformis) were popular writing material. The north Indian scholars used a thin layer of birch bark (*bhurjapatra*) to write. The *bhurjapatra* survives hardly few decades. So rewriting was an essential service to preserve thousands of manuscripts. The classics of medicine, *Caraka, Suśruta* and *Aṣṭānga samhitas* belong to this age of ayurveda. These three works are known as 'big three'.

Ayurveda in Brahminical Scriptures

Vedas, upavedas, araṇyakas, upaniṣads, and *purāṇas* provide innumerable references to medicine. However, they do not compete with 'big three' (*bṛhatrayī*) in dealing with health and disease so professionally. Vedas are the oldest reminiscences in the literary tradition of India. It is natural to think that the Vedic medicine is native to the Indian subcontinent. The word 'ayurveda' is not found in the Vedic literature. However, we find several references to diseases, medicines and causes of diseases in *Ṛgveda* and *Atharvaveda*. Vedas are divine for Hindus. They are venerated as sacred texts in archaic Sanskrit language inherited in oral tradition. The *Ṛgveda* is the oldest of them. The spells in the Vedas were devised for celebrations and various helpless situations. Some are praising the god and nature, some are blessings and some are curses. Some verses are for even to win in the wars and gambling. Vedic medicine is similar to occult medicine in other contemporary cultures. Most of the pragmatic therapies of the Vedic times have entered the treatises of ayurveda.

Study of Vedas and the medical lore of Europe establish links of Vedic culture to central Asian traditions. In essence, the Vedic medicine does not contain enough material that proves that it is the harbinger of ayurveda. Five element (*Pancamahābhuta*) theory, three humor (*tridoṣa*) theory, seven tissue (*saptadhātu*) theory etc are not found in the Vedic medical material.

Medicine and religion go together in early ages. The *Atharvaveda* (Veda of the fire-priests) hymns are not connected with the offering of *soma* in rituals. It consists chiefly of a variety of spells and incantations, intended to curse as well as to bless. The *Atharvaveda* is preserved in two recensions, comprising 730 hymns and about 6000 stanzas, spread in twenty books. Many of these verses are taken from *Ṛgveda* without change and some are in prose. These hymns provide clues to diseases that afflicted the Vedic people and near-contemporaries. Noteworthy part of the Vedas is their description of local flora as remedial in different diseases. While Ṛgveda reveals less of indigenous botanical knowledge, the Atharvaveda talks more of the local traditions and local flora.

Kenneth Zysk, the author of *Medicine in Veda*, opines that 'most likely the rivalry for power and prestige might have pushed the medical priests to lower strata of the society'. Medical priests are those who left the tradition of soma rituals and took medicine as profession. This led to a radical thinking in the medicine and subsequent development of principles of ayurveda. The differences between the Vedic medicine, which is magico-religious and the later empirico-rational medicine, ayurveda are obvious. The Vedic medicine believed in malevolent and benevolent spirits and deities that exist up above and cause good and bad on humans. The treatment consists of appeasing these spirits and deities. Ayurveda emphasizes on nature, balance among the humors in the body, diet and deed in preventing and curing the diseases. Although importance of physical factors was emphasized by ayurveda, it also admitted malevolent and benevolent spirits and deities as disease causing. Ayurveda has not yet shed its baggage on esoteric concepts in medicine. In pediatrics and obstetrics (the science of childbirth and diseases of newborn), the Vedic influence is still very strong.

Sanskrit scholars think *tridoṣa* theory has origins in the Atharvaveda. The word *vātīkṛta* occurs in Av 9.8.20. *Vāta* means wind and *kṛta* is becoming. There is another reference to the causes of death listing wind, water and fire. Bad wind blowing from any direction, apparently caused epidemics. Fire and water too are sources of disease and death. In the post-Vedic age, these three factors were considered as bodily entities. We breathe air incessantly and drink water frequently. As the fire (warmth), wind (moving air) and water constitute the universe and protect life on earth, the body was considered as a replica of the cosmos. The balance among these three factors is life and health. Ayurveda named them *vāta, pitta* and *kapha. Śleṣma* is a synonym for *kapha*. The word *dhātu* was used to denote these entities in the beginning. The word *doṣa* replaced *dhātu* some time later.

The diseases that were seriously affecting the people in the Vedic times were, *yakṣma* (consumption, tuberculosis), *jayanya* (a type of skin ulcer), *hṛdroga* (chest pain), *hariman* (jaundice), *balasa* (swelling), *takman* (various fevers), *kāsa* (cough), *rapas* (fragility and sickness), *viṣkanda-samskandha* (tetanus), *jalōdara* (ascites), *unmāda* (insanity), *krimi* (worms), *kilāsa* (discouloration of skin, leucoderma), and many other surgical complications due to accidents and blood loss. All these diseases are dealt in two ways: praying to the gods with established rituals and application of herbal medicines in various forms.

The contents of *Atharvaveda* clearly suggest that it was compiled many centuries after the *Rigveda*, to serve the local needs and contemporary problems in the Indian subcontinent. For instance, the word *krimi* (tiny or invisible insects and worms) does not appear in *Rigveda*, but the *Athavaveda* (2.31, 2.32, 5.23) talks about *krimi* elaborately. Varieties of names are given to them: *kururu, algandu, saluna, avaskava, vyadhvara, yevasha, kaskasa, ejatka* etc.

We find charms in Av 4.12; 5.5 against broken bones and wounds. The charms to cure flesh wounds and bleeding are found in Av 2.3; 6.44; 6.109. Therefore, the esoteric part of ayurveda is derived from Atharvaveda. Apparently, the content of Av is akin to the environment of the subcontinent. For instance, the name of *kapitha* (wood apple) tree appears in Atharvaveda but not in Rigveda. Many surgical techniques have roots in the *Atharvaveda*. In the condition of retention of urine, a primitive reed is inserted in to the urethra, the opening through which the urine is emptied, to facilitate urine excretion. In the later times, a sturdy metal catheter was introduced. The verses in *Av* 1.3 describe this technique of using a catheter.

Upaniṣads and Purāṇas

The upaniṣads are recordings of discourses on Vedic topics. They are derived from the Vedas by specific application of teachings of Vedas. *Manḍukya upaniṣad* talks about souls, self and the magical sound *aum*. *Kenopaniṣad* discusses and tries to define *brahma*. For instance, it says thinking mind is not brahma but by which the mind thinks is brahma! *Kaṭhopaniṣad* dwells into the meaning of life and death. In spite of abundant philosophical material in the upaniṣads, mundane world is intentionally disregarded and all upaniṣads see a purpose behind the creation and cosmos. Curious Hindu mind has interpreted the nature and consciousness in unending discourses.

Purāṇa is a form of historical record of facts blended with fantasy created in Sanskrit language during the Gupta Empire between 4th and 6th centuries AD. In 18th and 19th centuries, historians have not counted on these chronicles as a source of history. However, the *purāṇas* undoubtedly give some important information on historical facts. *Purāṇa* is a story based on historical events woven into fantasy. Each *purāṇa* narrates a story conveying a moral code or salvation. Although the number of *purāṇas* runs beyond one hundred, there are 18 *purāṇas* which are valid and authored at least one thousand years ago. All of the 18 (*aṣṭadaśa*) *purāṇas* are thought to be authored by Vyasa. Many *purāṇas* were created during the medieval period. *Linga purāṇa, Vāyu purāṇa, Viṣnu purāṇa, Bhagavāta purāṇa* and *Garuḍa purāṇa* contain some ideas on treatment, diseases, longevity and growth of life in the womb. *Agnipurāṇa* accolades Dhanvantari recommending several herbal prescriptions to get healed or to live longer. In the voice of Dhanvatari ways to revive the dead are pronounced. Most of the data in these scriptures is fantastic. *Garuḍa purāṇa* exclusively deals with origin of life and several diseases like leprosy and tuberculosis. The *Bhāgavata purāṇa* narrates the story of Parikshist maharaj, who was cursed by the sun and seeking a guru's teaching. Suta Gosvami accidentally meets Parikshit and enlightens him by his teaching. Their discourses are described in the *purāṇa.* The *Bhagavāta purāṇa* describes evolution, *pancabhuta, triguṇa* (three psychic humors) and Dhanvantari. It also narrates an incident of Aśvini twins joining the severed head with torso. Time dilation theory too was guessed in *Bhāgavata purāṇa.* Kakudni and Revati go to *brahmalōka* (heaven) and return to this mundane world and find all their contemporaries are dead! This occurrence is often compared to 'time warp' theory.

Some *purāṇas* yield actual information on some historical events. Major difference between an ayurveda treatise like *Carakasamhita* and a *purāṇa* like *Garuda purāṇa* is obvious. *Purāṇas* emphasize on magical cures and no explanation is found on the drug action. *Puraṇas* insist on diseases caused by sin. The ayurveda treatises try to emphasize on the empirical and rational elements of medicine because they were composed by professional physicians. *Purāṇas* were composed by the scholars other than physicians. Obviously, ayurveda treatises were composed by Buddhists scholars, who collected nectar from the religious literature and rendered it secular to serve the public. Today's ayurveda physician is not properly trained on content and importance of Vedas, upaniṣads and purāṇas and their role in the evolution of ayurveda.

In the 19th century Horace Hayman Wilson (1786 - 1860) made a systematic study of *puraṇas* and translated *Viṣnu purāṇa* in to English with a critical commentary. H.H. Wilson was also interested in ayurveda. He was an active member of the Medical and Physical Society of Bengal, which published a journal on contemporary medicine in India.

Darśana or Indian Philosophy

Philosophy is the mother of all sciences, whether it was in ancient Greece or India. Observation, reasoning and philosophical debates in ancient Greece led to some disciplines of science like geometry, astronomy, medicine and life sciences. In India, debates and discourses on epistemological methods and *self* versus *nature* have created a rich heritage of psychological insights in philosophical thought. The basic principles of ayurveda are derived from three philosophical systems of ancient India, *Sānkhya, Nyāya* and *Vaiśeṣika darśanas*. The remaining *darśanas, Yōga, Vedanta* and *Mimāmsa* too played a vital role in sanskritizing the medical knowledge of ancient India.

The word *darśana* means vision. An outlook

of a thinker on matter and life is narrated in *darśana*. An ancient Indian saying tells each mind has its own philosophy. However, the views of influential thinkers of ancient India have been grossly divided into six *darśanas*. Some other schools of philosophy representing atheists and rationalists (nāstika, ajivika, Jaina and Buddha) were later ignored. In fact, sixteen different patterns are identified in the philosophical tradition of India. The speculations advocated in *darśanas* are much older than the *darśanas* themselves. Vedas are a collection of sacrificial rituals and apprehensions of humankind but *darśanas* reveal psychological erudition and evolution of ideas. The influence of six philosophical systems (*ṣaḍ-darśana*) is enormous on ayurveda. The medical knowledge collated from different sources was housed in a framework provided by six *darśanas*. These systems and their propounded / reformed by…

1. *SānkhyaDarśana* – propounded by Kapila
2. *Vaiśeṣika Darśana* – propounded by Kanada
3. *YōgaDarśana* – systematized by Patanjali
4. *NyāyaDarśana* – founded by Gautama
5. *Mīmāmsa Darśana* – advocated by Jaimini
6. *Vedānta Darśana* – synthesized by Badarayana

Sānkhya Darśana of Kapila advocates that nothing can be created out of void. It advocates dualism i.e. *puruṣa* (soul of self) and *prakṛti* (nature) as two different products or entities. *Puruṣa* is self or awareness. The *puruṣa* is multiple too. The *prakṛti* with its three characters *satva, rajas* and *tama*, evolves and imbibe *puruṣa*. The universe including *puruṣa* is an evolutionary product. It looks at the human body resembling a microcosm or mini-model of the universe. The *prakṛti* is held to have two distinctive states, quiescent and emergent. In the quiescent state, constituent traits (*guṇas*) are in a state of *sāmya* or dynamic equilibrium; in the emergent they are in a state of *vaiṣamya* or instability, which drives them to clash, and cooperate and strive for ascendancy.

The *avyakta* (un-manifested) is manifested into *mahat* (manifested), which in turn originates *ahamkāra* (body-less soul) with three characteristics namely *satva, rajas* and *tamas,* which can be translated into pleasure, pain and delusions. Later, *pancatanmātra* (five subtle elements) are born. All these eight categories are known as *aṣthaprakṛti*. This gave rise to *ṣoḍaśa vikriti* (sixteen derivatives). They are *pancamahābhuta* (five gross elements), *pancajnānendriya* (five sensory organs – *akṣi* (eye), *nāsa* (nose), *jihva* (tongue), *karṇa* (ear) and *tvaca* (skin)), *pancakarmendriya* (five motor organs – *vāk* (larynx-speech), *hasta* (hand-doing), *pāda* (foot-mobility), *pāyu* (anus-excretion) and *upastha* (vagina-reproduction) and *manas* (mind)). All these twenty four elements together are known as *caturvimśati tatva* (24 entities). Ayurveda treatises concede to this idea of *caturvimśati tatva puruṣa*.

Sānkhya accepts only three modalities as sources of knowledge, *pratyakṣa* (direct evidence), *anumāna* (inference) and *āptavākya* (testimony). Ayurveda has taken *yukti*, a form of syllogism as a source of knowledge. Kapila is the foremost philosopher of India. However, it was over-emphasized that Kapila is the only philosopher in India and Sānkhya is the only philosophy! (*ekmeva darśanam, sānkhyameva darśanam*). Kapila preceded Gowthama Buddha, who learned some Sāmkhya principles from Ārāḍha.

Kanada's *Vaiśeṣika darśana* advocates atomic theory to understand the structure and function of universe. Kanada was said to be collecting granules, seeds and other edible tree products from the forest floor to sustain, hence the name kan-ada, eater of granules. The word *Vaiśeṣika* means particularity. *Vaiśeṣika darśana* looks at the nature as objective and independent of the observer. Kanada identifies seventeen *guṇas* (traits) like color, smell etc coexisting with matter. Because of several later commentaries and additions, it is difficult to isolate the mind of Kanada from other commentators. The atomic theory of ancient Greece is close to this concept. The Jains venerate Kanada. It advocates perception and inference alone help acquire knowledge. This system is a theistic form of atomism.

Gautama's *Nyāya darśana* (*Nyāyasutra*) played an important role in creating epistemological base for ayurveda. The logic of *Nyaya darśana* was built upon the ideas of Akshapāda Gotama. The *Carakasamhita* alludes several times to the logic borrowed from the *Nyāya darśana* to substantiate its concepts. It accepts direct evidence (*pratyakṣa*), inference (*anumāna*), conjunction (*yukti*) and testimony(*āptavākya*) as ways and means of getting knowledge.

Patanjali's *Yōga darśana* has influenced the concepts of ayurveda in *manōvijnāna,* (psychology and psychiatry) and parapsychology. After the decline of Buddhism in India, ayurveda classics turned to Jaimini's *Mimāmsa* and Badarayana's *Vedānta darśanas* to reinterpret the concepts of ayurveda to suit the changing cultural and religious scenario. Pyrrhon of Elis from Greece accompanied Alexander to India in the 4th century BC and was influenced by *mimamsa* philosophy, who in turn introduced it to the west. The dominant philosophical schools of India strongly believed in material-spiritual disjunction. Those who decline the eternal existence of *ātma* (soul) are branded as atheists and enemies of ayurveda. *Mīmāmsa darśana* is also known as *purva mīmāmsa* and *Vedanta darśana* is known as *uttara mīmāmsa*. They take testimony (*āptavākya*) as valid and valuable way of knowing truth. The direct evidence, and inference, according to *mimāmsa*, may mislead us to misunderstanding. The believers of this system ignore the fact that the testimony (*āptavākya*) too was derived from direct or indirect evidence by our predecessors. *Vedānta* literally means end of the Veda or Veda-end. It influenced the philosophy of ayurveda more than any other school of thought from the middle Ages did. It gave utmost importance to the *āptavākya* in validating the theories and concepts.

Origins of Ayurveda

The origin of ayurveda is shrouded in unexplored history. We do not know exactly when the word ayurveda came into usage. It is a new bottle for the old wine. Several fables were crafted around origins of ayurveda during the last two thousand years. The treatises are unanimous in proposing finite nature to human knowledge about medicine. It is believed that the nectar of ayurveda was salvaged by the god Dhanvantari from the churning of ocean. This knowledge is transmitted to the sages to serve the humankind. The knowledge and wisdom of ayurveda is packaged in 100,000 Sanskrit stanzas arranged in one thousand chapters. Several ayurveda physicians believe that new additions to ayurveda are merely a rediscovery of the forgotten parts of the original compositions.

Historians of ayurveda in the West see a break between Vedic medicine and ayurveda, because several elements of ayurveda do not have seeds in Vedas. Historians of ayurveda in India do not accept or tolerate break in medical ideology between Vedic and post-Vedic periods, but rather strongly believe in continuity from Veda to ayurveda. Hindu divinities are believed to be the ultimate fountains from which the knowledge and wisdom of ayurveda originated.

According to *Carakasamhita* (1.2-40) Brahma, the supreme god, has passed on the knowledge of ayurveda to Prajapati and he in turn taught Aśvini twins. The Aśvini twins are legendary healers, from whom Bharadvaja learned ayurveda. Suddenly new name appears here: Punarvasu Ātreya. He teaches ayurveda to six disciples Aginveśa, Bhela, Jatukarṇa, Parāśara, Kṣārapāṇi and Hārita. But who taught ayurveda to Ātreya? Cakrapāṇi, the 12thcentury commentator on *Carakasamhita*, thinks Indra taught to Bharadvāja and Atri, in turn Atri taught it to Ātreya. The commentators and redactors have skillfully constructed the mythologies to give an impression that ayurveda is a Hindu science since its inception.

Suśrutasamhita (1.1-21) gives another story. Brahma taught ayurveda to Prajapati, who taught Aśvins. Indra learned ayurveda from Aśvini twins, who indoctrinated Dhanvantari to ayurveda. Suśruta was the student of Dhanvantari. *Aṣṭāngahṛdaya* (a little older than *Sangraha*) gives slightly a different lineage. Brahma reveals ayurveda to Prajapati from whom Aśvins twins learn. Indra garnered the knowledge from Aśvins. The sages Dhanvantari, Bharadvaja, Nimi, and Kaśyapa approached Punarvasu Ātreya to be their leader to request revelation from Indra. However, *Aṣṭāngahṛdaya* closely supports Caraka's view of origin.

It is assumed by all redactors and commentators that ayurveda is a subdivision of the Atharvaveda. Ayurveda was composed in one hundred thousand verses, and arranged into one thousand chapters by Lord Brahma before he created the world. However, because of the short life span and limited intellectual capacity of humans, Dhanvantari reduced ayurveda to eight parts, viz. major surgery (*śalya*), supraclavical surgery (*śalākya*), general medicine (*kāyacikitsa*), demonology (*bhutavidya*), pediatrics and obstetrics (*kaumārabhṛtya*), toxicology (*agadatantra*), use of organic elixirs (*rasāyanatantra*), and the science of fertility and virility (*Vājikaraṇatantra*). These are the classical eight limbs (*angas*) of ayurveda.

During the *Brāhmana* and *Upaniṣad* periods (c.700 B.C.) only four branches of ayurveda, namely *Bhutavidya, Sarpavidya* (healing snakebite), *Rasāyana* and *Vājikaraṇa* were recorded. *Kāyacikitsa* (internal medicine), *Śalya* (General Surgery), *Śalākya* (Ear, Nose, Throat, Dental and Ophthalmology) and *Kaumārabhṛtya* (Pediatrics) were added later. Finally, ayurveda became *Aṣṭānga* (eight branched) ayurveda. However, the growth of ayurveda is clearly visible during the last 20-30 centuries. Ayurveda compositions of the Middle Ages added several new diseases and medicinal formulations not discussed earlier in the treatises. In fact, a detailed table of names of diseases and symptoms will unravel the entry of new diseases and drugs through the ages. From the Vedic period up to the modern age, ayurveda had undergone several changes. This evolution is clearly visible.

Rasāyana cikitsa aims at procrastinating geriatric problems in the old age. *Vājikaraṇa cikitsa* is intended to give birth to healthy babies. Surprisingly, the branch of *Vājikaraṇa* is very ancient in ayurveda. It is one of the eight branches of ayurveda. *Vāji* in Sanskrit means horse. It is often overemphasized that *Vājikaraṇa* is a process to enhance virility in men. It is a common belief in India that horse is the most virile animal. Observation of wild horses in central Asia yielded interesting information. Wild horses live in groups of 8 or 9. The stallion, the dominant male horse, has more chances of copulation with female horses. So the offspring is always more healthy. Horses emerge more powerful as the generations pass by. This idea was depicted in the word *Vājikaraṇa*. Caraka points out to the health of the to-be-born children as the goal of *Vājikaraṇa*. However, many ayurveda physicians claim today that *Vājikaraṇa* is to enhance the pleasures of sex.

Dynamics of Ayurveda

The essence of ayurveda lies in the comprehension of attributes of matter (*gurvādi guṇa*). The qualities or attributes are inherent and inseparable from the matter. Nature of the nature lies in these traits. The *puruṣa* (human body), is considered as a microcosm of the universe. All animate and inanimate beings inevitably contain flavor (*rasa*), property (*guṇa*) and potency (*vīrya*). Caraka extolled *...there is no substance in the universe which cannot be used as drug on the condition that they are used rationally and with definite objective.*

These attributes are twenty in number. The technique of imparting these qualities in an individual is one of the protocols of ayurveda therapy. This entails the principle of similarities; i.e., similarities cause increase while dissimilarities cause decrease. Hot quality in the environment or diet will increase hotness in the body. A food item considered to be heavy will make the body heavier. In all cultures believe in the concept of hot and cool states of the body. When sleep is inadequate, a burning sensation in the stomach, feeling burning sensation while urinating etc. are understood as symptoms of hot body. Common cold, cough etc indicate the opposite. People think the ingredients of the food are responsible for it.

The idea of *guṇa* (attributes) in ayurveda has been borrowed from the *Nyāya darśana*. The qualities attributed to the matter are:

1. *Guru* (heavy) – *Laghu* (light)
2. *Manda* (slow) – *Tikṣṇa* (quick, sharp)
3. *Hima* (cold) – *Uṣṇa* (hot)
4. *Snigdha* (unctuous) – *Rukṣa* (dry)
5. *Slakṣṇa* (smooth) – *Khara* (rough)
6. *Sāndra* (solid) – *Drava* (liquid)
7. *Mṛdu* (soft) – *Kaṭhina* (hard)
8. *Sthira* (stable) – *Cala* (mobile)
9. *Sukṣma* (subtle) – *Sthula* (gross)
10. *Viṣada* (non-slimy) – *Picchila* (slimy)

All beings, both animate and inanimate,

possess combination of these ten pairs of attributes to some degree. Each pair of traits refers to only one characteristic because they are relative to each other. Hot and cold, solid and liquid, soft and hard so on so forth. Food imparts these qualities gradually in to the human body, while the medicine transfers these attributes to the body instantaneously. The traits of matter can be interpreted after consuming the substance in edible form and note the changes in bodily phenomena and psychic feelings. Most of this knowledge is subjective. Therefore, there is a big scope for difference of opinion. All sweet substances invariably contain carbohydrates and thus superfluous glucose turns fat and increase body weight. Therefore, ayurveda theorizes *madhura* (sweet) substances increase body weight (*guru*). The bitter substances accordingly decrease body weight. It can be further inferred that sweet flavor (*madhura rasa*) stimulates humor phlegm (*kapha doṣa*) and pungent flavor (*kaṭu rasa*) stimulates humor wind (*vāta doṣa*).

Before attempting to alter the attributes (*guṇa*), the physician has to be conscious of the predisposition of the body, i.e. *Prakṛti* (constitution). The constitution of the body is inherited from several sources like father (*pitrujanya*), mother (*matrujanya*), nutrition (*poṣana*), self (*ātmaja*) temporal (*kālaja*) etc. The constitution/temperament inherited cannot be changed during the lifetime. The domination of any of the three humors (*vāta, pitta* and *kapha*) makes the person more susceptible to certain diseases in different seasons.

Every physical or psychological indulgence too can vitiate the humors. The factors that vitiate the humors are basically three in number *viz.*. *indriya-indriyārtha sannikarṣa* (interaction of the sensory organs with the nature), *prajñāparādha* (fallacy) and *pariṇāma* (seasonal changes). When the sensory organs are misused or exposed to inappropriate sensations like looking at too much brightness or staying in the dark for long time, listening to louder noises etc., any of the *doṣas* (humors) get vitiated leading to diseases in the long run. Fallacy is a kind of psychological indulgence or enslaving oneself to bad habits like binge drinking and smoking, disrespect to nature etc. *Pariṇāma* (variations according to climate and seasons) is another important natural cause of the disease. If the recommended seasonal regimen is ignored, the human being becomes susceptible to disease. However, some diseases may be caused by *karma* (past actions).

According to the ancient *Sānkhya* theory of cosmogony, on which Ayurveda is based, the 'five proto elements' (*pancamahābhuta*) combine in different proportions to form the material world. Each element possesses different amounts of the above-mentioned *guṇas*; thus, each element has its unique qualitative nature. The elements are:

1. *Akāśa* – space
2. *Vāyu* – air

3. *Agni* or *tejas* – fire
4. *Ap* or *jala* – water
5. *Prithvi* or *bhumi* – earth

The concept of humors is ubiquitous across several civilizations. Hellenistic and Chinese traditions too believe in the concept of 'cardinal humors'. Ayurveda believes that three humors (*tridoṣa*) *vāta*, *pitta* and *kapha* govern all bodily processes. The general reading of hymns related to medicine in the Atharvaveda gives a general idea that the fire, water and wind as the causative factors of disease and death. The wind, fire and water are indispensable tools for the human life. These are the homologues of *vāta, pitta* and *kapha/sleṣma* inside the human body. These three humors are on constant fluctuation depending on season, time of the day, age, sex, diet and deed. However, human being is endowed with a domination of one of three humors since the birth. This predomination of one or two humors influences the person's behavior and health. This is known as a constitution type. Each constitution type has particular strengths and susceptibilities, according to the principles of ayurveda.

Ayurveda scholars are reluctant to respond to the question 'whether the *doṣas* are tangible or intangible'. This question is immaterial for them. The description in the *Carakasamhita* is clear that the *doṣas* are material in nature. Initially the word *dhātu* (constituent) was used to denote *doṣa*. The traits of *vāta* are described by Vagbhata as '*tatra rukṣo laghussitaha kharasukṣma scaloanilaha*' (dry, light, cool, rough, fine, mobile), *pitta* as *sasneha tikṣnokṣam laghu visram saram dravam* (oily, sharp, hot, light, smelly, flowing, liquid) *kapha* as *snigdhassito gururmandaha slakṣṇo mṛtsnaha sthira kapha* (oily, cool, heavy, slow, sticky, smelly, stable). These qualities are physical and tangible. Today's scholars turned to the concept of invisibility of *doṣas*.

The modern science has dissected the human body and shown us the real structure. Ayurveda philosophers seek a way out and ascribe new meanings to old words. They stretch their imagination to justify their notions. All traditional systems of medicine depend on physical attributes of matter for interpretation. The chemical structure of the matter determines its physical properties. Therefore, depending on physical traits may also lead us truth but there are limitations to it.

The ayurvedic practitioner will have to assess the signs and symptoms of a disease, the patient's unique *prakṛti*, and *samprāpti* (pathogenesis) to arrive at a treatment plan. The treatment schedule will consist of using herbs and prescribing *pathyāpathya* (changes in the diet). All the medicinal herbs are screened for their *rasa* (flavour), *guṇa* (attributes), *vīrya* (potency), *vipāka* (post-digestive assimilation) and *prabhāva* (special effect). Any herbal raw product sweet in taste is taken as pacifying *kapha doṣa* and increasing body weight. Bitter substances decrease body weight and promote *vāta doṣa*. When this logic is not sufficient to interpret the drug action, special effect (*prabhāva*) is considered. Therefore, the *prabhāva* is an axiom beyond interpretation. Thus, ayurveda is empirico-rational medicine. The utility of a drug or diet is assessed only after its prolonged use on the patients and the *guṇa, vīrya, vipāka* and *prabhāva* are standardized. Chakrapani of 12th century A.D. says 'inherent nature (*svabhāva*) of the elements is such that one cannot predict which properties will become manifest in a particular mixture of the elements because the choice of these properties is governed by the force of the invisible (*adṛṣṭaprabhāva*).

The Big Three

The *Aṣṭāngahṛdaya* is a major work authored by Vagbhata, who resided in Sindhudesa, a province in present-day Pakistan. It is considered as quintessence of both *Carakasamhita* and *Suśrutasamhita*. A Chinese pilgrim, I-Tsing, who travelled in India between 672 AD and 688 AD, tells that this treatise is recently composed and all the physicians in five parts of India practice according to this book.

The *Carakasamhita* was originally authored by the sage Aginveśa, probably between 800 B.C. and 500 B.C. Caraka has redacted the *Aginveśasamhita*. Historians have identified Caraka as the personal physician of the Kushan king Kaniska in the 2nd c. B.C. The *Carakasamhita* was later re-edited by Driḍabala, a Kashmiri scholar in the 2nd c. AD. The *Suśrutasamhita* represents the Dhanvantari school of medicine. It was composed by Suśruta, well known creative surgeon of ancient India. Suśruta elaborately deals with the surgical problems, hence, it is considered as a prime textbook of surgery in ayurveda. A scholar by name Nagarjuna has redacted it and added several chapters at the end, known as *Uttaratantra*. Suśruta has described several surgical operations *viz.* Removing stones from urinary tracts, Cesarean operation to bring out the unborn baby in emergencies, rhinoplasty (a technique to reconstruct the lost nose from skin of forehead), several techniques of bandages in fractures of bones and suturing split wounds. Most of these techniques are similar to the modern methods except for the fact that the absence of anesthesia had tested the time of the unfortunate patients and surgeons. These three works, *Carakasamhita, Suśrutasamhita* and *Aṣṭāngahṛdaya* are known as *bṛhatrayi*, the Great Three or Big Three. The treatises, Caraka and Suṣruta are not popular in South India until the colonial times!

It is beyond dispute that the original *Aginveśasamhia* was not handed down because there was no script at the time of its appearance. All the treatises appeared in script only after the first century AD. The habit of Indian scholars is different from the western scholars. We still can read Homer's Iliad or Megasthanes Indica in unaltered form. In India, the scholars always meddled in intellectual blasphemy. Instead of attempting to redact Aginveśasamhita, why Caraka hasn't tried to write his own treatise? Historians of medicine now depend on commentaries and redacted versions to upgrade or justify the outdated concepts. Today, it is difficult to see the original mind of initial writers because of commentaries and additions. This habit has fossilized the knowledge. Moreover, this practice has altered our perceptions. Vaghbata was certainly a Buddhist. The references to prove this fact were wiped out by ensuing writers. However, some manuscripts of *Aṣṭāngasangraha*, available in some libraries across India pay homage to Buddha. In the manuscripts commented by Indu these changes happened.

Fortunately, some manuscripts recovered unaltered from 4th and 5th centuries, provide us with a fresh look at medicine 1500 years ago in India. The Bower's manuscript, which became known at the end of 19th century, was scripted by Buddhist monks, recovered by a British officer Bower, and now preserved in Oxford, England. This is the oldest manuscript of ayurveda available today.

Climate and Seasons

Climate played an important role in the formation of principles of ayurveda. The recommended daily and seasonal regimen is the cornerstone to prevent diseases and enjoy good health. The balance among three humors is highly dependent on various elements like temperature, rainfall, dietary habits, age, time of the day etc. Therefore, the climate and weather influence the level of humors in the body. Any long-lasting imbalance leads to disease. The seasons and their influences are discussed at length in all the treatises of ayurveda.

The tropic of Cancer divides India into northern temperate zone and southern tropical zone. The sun shifts between the imagined lines of Cancer and Capricorn year-round. The Sun's northern and southern sojourns are known as *uttarāyana* and *dakṣiṇāyana* respectively. Any place beyond the tropic of Cancer in north India, experiences sun's maximum culmination only once a year (23rd June). Any location on any latitude in South India will observe the sun moving from south to further north, and back every year, because south India lies from 8^0 N to equator and extend up to 21^0 N. South India lies in tropical zone. North India lies in subtropical zone. Hence, the sun crosses overhead in all locations of south India *twice* a year. This phenomenon does not happen in northern India. The tilt of the earth on its axis rather than the movement of the sun on the horizon cause the *uttarāyana* (path to the north) and *dakṣināyana* (path to the south). The commencement of *dakṣināyana* (23rd June) is same everywhere in north India. For south Indians, *dakṣināyana* exhibits very different climate.

Tradition in India reckons six seasons in a year, two months each. The Indian subcontinent, with east-west extension of 3000 k.m. and north-south extension of similar distance, experiences seasons in different regions with some interval. These seasons vary slightly from one region to the other, especially from Kashmir to Kerala. However, these variations are not discussed in the treatises of ayurveda. The climate of the south is different from the north, because the subcontinent is divided by the tropic of Cancer into tropical and subtropical regions. Many of the therapeutic measures described in ayurveda are suitable to the subtropical climates. Ayurveda physicians of South India have not appropriated the daily and seasonal regimen to suit the climate in South India.

The average annual rainfall in south India is less than 200 c.m. per annum. Most of the rain is received from the 'southwest' monsoon in the months of June, July and August. Sahyadri mountain range receives lion's share during this season. Sometimes, the monsoon starts in May and continues up to September. The 'northeast' monsoon showers over the southeastern part of India in November and December. The southwest monsoon first touches the Malabar Coast in May-June; therefore, West Coast gets intense rainfall during this period. This region is known for spices. The typical topography of Kerala with its high temperatures, humidity, good rainfall and hilly slopes the pepper plants grow wild. This plant needs good rain for pollination.

The zone east to the Western Ghats or Sahyadri mountain range receives leftover rainfall. The monsoon clouds hover over the subcontinent for 4 months in two branches, one entering over Malabar Coast and other over the Bay of Bengal because the Arakoan Mountains in Myanmar divert this cloud over to India. Therefore, the monsoon starts in May and continues until September. However, no place in India receives rain in all these months. The east coast is battered by cyclones frequently, as the Bay of Bengal is a favorable breeding ground for the series of cyclones in the summer and fall.

Vagbhata says 'the *uttarayana* (sun's northern sojourn) debilitates the human body while the *dakṣināyana* strengthens it'. So, measures that are more preventive are recommended for the winter and spring. More curative measures are recommended for the summer and rainy seasons. This concept is obviously applicable to the people residing in northern subtropics but not entirely applicable to the people living in the tropics, because the time of the commencement of *dakṣināyana* is much later in South India. The *hemanta ritu* (winter) is different from north to south.

The description of six seasons in *Suśrutasamhita* (*sutrasthāna* 4th chapter) is slightly different; it says *Varṣaśaradhemanta vasantagrīṣmaprāvṛṭ ṣadritavo bhavanti*...this quotation does not refer to the *śiśira* (cold), but adds *pravṛṭ ṛtu* between *grīṣma* and *varṣa*. *Pravṛṭ* season corresponds to *āṣāḍa* and *śrāvaṇa* (June and July) months. The rainy season according to this statement is August and September. The southwest monsoon reaches the northwest part of India in mid August and continues into September. The *Carakasamhita* talks about six seasons *viz.. śiśira, vasanta, grīṣma, varṣa, sarad and hemanta* in the 6th chapter of *Sutrasthana*. These observations explain the local variations of climate.

In spite of these differences, the treatises are unanimous in accepting the importance of only three seasons: summer, monsoon/rainy and winter, because only these three seasons show strong impact on health and disease. These seasonal variations deflect the humors. Physiology turns to pathology if the deflection of humors is not set right.

Caraka and Vagbhata talk about *sancaya* (aggregation), *prakōpa* (vitiation) and *praśamana* (pacification) of the humors, *vāta, pitta* and *kapha* in *grīṣma* (summer), *varṣa* (rainy season) and *hemanta* (winter) respectively - each stage lasting about 2 months. Ayurveda believed in the alternating seasonal impact on the human body. They aggravate in the ensuing season and pacify in the next in normal condition. If the seasonal regimen is ignored the humor, instead of being pacified further aggravates and causes disease.

Suśruta describes *kriyākāla*, six pathological stages of the diseases instead of three stages of humors like Caraka. These six stages arc not related to the seasons but to the state of the pathology or disease-process in the body. The first and second stages may be triggered by the changing climates. The rise or vitiation of the particular *doṣa* or humor causes certain diseases. Accordingly, ayurveda prescribes suitable diet and deed for each season to stay healthy. This is the first indication of rational approach to medicine. Due to diverse geographical locations in India, the recommendations of ayurveda to prevent diseases need correction to suit other latitudes.

The coastal plains with swampy regions are a good breeding ground for the mosquitoes and the people suffer from several diseases like malaria, filariasis, giardiasis etc. Suśruta, for the first time in the history of medicine, links the prevalence of *slīpada* (elephantiasis) to the swampy regions, where mosquitoes can breed and spread the disease. Although Suśruta could not predict mosquito as causative factor for the disease, he could draw his attention to swampy regions where water is stagnant and favorable to diseases like *slīpada.* The *Mādhavanidāna,* a 1200-year-old prime textbook of pathology, also corroborates this view.

Ayurveda recommends the use of herbs locally grown to treat the diseases. In each ecosystem humans and plants, establish a natural rhythm to each other. The winter and summer idylls recommended in the texts of ayurveda do not show any inhibitions. The life in ancient India was tuned to vagaries of seasons.

Ayurveda and Buddhism

Religion and science are fruits of philosophy. Indian philosophy gave birth to more than one religion, among them Buddhism is the most erudite and benevolent. Buddhism was a dominant faith in India for more than 1500 years. It also helped catalyze the Vedic beliefs and practices to more refined form. Buddhist families in ancient India have voluntarily conscripted at least one son from their families to Buddhist clergy. The ordained monks were trained in religion, logic, ethics and medicine. Buddhist monks were always on the move, except during the rainy season, to meet new people. *Stupa* (mound or relic), *vihāra* (monastery) and *caitya* (place for worship) are well known structures in Buddhist architecture. Ascetics spend monsoon season in a *vihāra*, which is a dormitory for housing monks. *Vihāras* are found in picturesque locations throughout India. They were built in bricks or carved out of stone. The name of province Bihar, comes from this word, where *vihāras* were built abundantly and monks used to roam the land in great numbers. The other meaning of *vihāra* is 'to roam'. *Stupa* is a round and tall structure built to conceal a casket holding a bone fragment or tooth of Buddha. Amaravati, Sanchi and Dhamek (Saranath) *Stupas* are few examples of such structures. Buddhists go round these *Stupas* in folded hands several times to pay respect to Buddha. *Caitya* is an assembly hall for prayer. The patients, old and infirm people flocked to hospices, organized by Buddhist *sangha* in several parts of India. They were the public hospitals in ancient India.

Buddhism was a social movement against the unjust Vedic society. It is an organized reconstruction of the society. It fought against caste discrimination, gender discrimination and inhuman tendencies of dominant social groups in the society. It also encouraged systematization of knowledge using peoples' languages like *pali* and *prakrit.* Gautama Buddha discounted Sanskrit as a useful media to spread the word of dharma. The literature in vernacular languages was more voluminous than in Sanskrit but unfortunately India has lost most of this treasure. This has been big loss to the people of India. Sadly enough, the scholars of ayurveda in

India forget the contributions of Buddhism in systematizing the medical lore.

By the time of Buddha in the 6th century BC, physicians in Takshasila used to teach medicine to students, who come in search of famous teachers. Takshasila in northwest India was an important centre for ayurveda. The existence of a renowned physician Jivaka in Rajagriha is confirmed by the Buddhist literature. Jivaka went to Takshasila to study medicine. Atreya was his teacher. There is a famous story about the final examination Jivaka had undergone. Jivaka was asked to identify any plant, which is not useful in medicine. After roaming the surroundings of Takshasila, Jivaka could not find any herb, which is useless, and therefore, Jivaka graduated from Takshasila. His teacher gave him some money for travel expenses when Jivaka departed to Rajagriha. En route, money was exhausted. In a town Saketa, Jivaka used his knowledge and cured a chronic disease of a rich merchant's wife and earned money. He proceeded to Rajagriha, where he became a legendary physician. The emperor of Magadha, Bimbisara was suffering from fistula-in-ano and Jivaka could cure him. He rendered medical services to Gautama Buddha too. According to *Mahavagga* (a section of *Vinayapiṭaka*) Jivaka performed several surgical operations. One of them is opening the abdomen and 'disentangling twisted intestines' of a person! Jivaka treated king Pejjota of Ujjain, who was suffering from jaundice with medicated ghee. The king was averse to take ghee but after taking medicine got relieved of his problem. The treatise written by Jivaka has perished in the ravages of time. Some surgical treatments described in the Buddhist literature were certainly fabricated fables over a period.

If ayurveda was already in such a matured state by the time of Buddha, what is the contribution of Buddhism to ayurveda? Archaeological excavations in Taksasila, present day Taxila in Pakistan, did not yield any valid proof of existence of university there, although some famous people like Chanakya, Patanjali, Mahali of Vaisali, Pasendi of Kosala studied there. In the 6th, 5th centuries BC, Takshasila was a famous educational centre but without any formal university, classrooms etc. For nearly one thousand years, the city of Takshasila existed successively at three sites – Bhir mound, Sirkap and Sirsukh, representing the ancient, Greek and Kushana phases of political history. All three places have been extensively excavated, but archaeologists have not found evidences of university campus. Therefore, the historians assume that the teachers used to host the students at home and teach. Later, a number of Buddhist monasteries were built at Takshasila and they became seats of learning.

Buddhism spread to other parts of Asia, Middle East including Egypt when proselyte Asoka converted to Buddhism in the 3rd century BC. Ayurveda spread to south India even before the ascendency of Asoka, the greatest Mauryan ruler. 33 inscriptions of Asoka, which are etched on big boulders (major rock edicts), minor rocks and pillars from across the entire subcontinent (India, Pakistan, Bangladesh and Nepal. These inscriptions talk about the medical facilities to be made. He recommends the import of medicinal plants where it is necessary and dispense medicines. In the group of Jonnagiri (Erragudi) inscriptions of Asoka in Andhra Pradesh, etched on rock boulders between the years 259 – 256 BC, the ninth pillar edict informs that the people, particularly women, perform several religious rites when sick. This indicates that the people depend on providence for health. The second pillar edict at Erragudi proclaims that hospitals for animals and human beings should be established and medicinal plants useful in treatment should be bought from other places and cultivated where they are not growing. The second pillar edict is a clear indication that medicinal plants locally available were not sufficient to meet the health care needs according to the prevailing knowledge of ayurveda in northern India. Therefore, the king has ordered for import and cultivation of medicinal plants.

Buddhism further spread into southern regions; into the kingdoms of Cola, Pandya and Cera. Cola and Pandya kingdoms were ruling Tamil speaking region and Cera in Malabar, present day Kerala. Asokan inscriptions are found in several places of north Karnataka – Sannati (Bijapur district), Maski (Raichur district), Siddhapura (Bellary district). Buddhist architecture is seen in Aihole and Badami, the erstwhile capitals of Calukyas in Karnataka more than 1500 years ago. Buddhist sculpture is also recovered at Hampi, the capital of Viajayanagara Empire.

Asoka's son, Mahindra, while taking Buddhism to Srilanka, popularized it in south India. Buddhism flourished in Kerala from 2nd century

B.C. to 8th century AD. Many Buddhists enjoyed royal patronage until 12th century AD. Buddhist temples were transformed into Hindu temples in ensuing years. Vadakkunathan temple of Thrissur, Kurumba Bhagawathi temple of Kannur and Durga temple at Paruvaserri near Thrissur in Kerala are few examples. Tamilnadu and Srilanka were deeply influenced by Buddhism. Kanchipuram, Srirnagapattana and Madurai were important Buddhist centers up to 7th century AD. However, from 7th century AD onwards Buddhism started declining in Tamilnadu. *Manimekalai* is a well-known work on Buddhism in Dravidadeśa.

Buddhism played an active role in the formation of concepts of ayurveda. The portions of medical lore collected by the wandering physicians were later codified by Buddhist monasteries. The symbiotic relationship between Buddhism and medicine has facilitated the spread of Buddhism in India. Monk-healers of many monasteries have attracted the sick and infirm people and served them in the hospices and infirmaries. Their selfless service has helped Buddhism to spread *Dhamma* and increase its influence on the society.

Medicine Buddha

There are umpteen numbers of references to medicine in *Tripiṭas*, the scriptures of Buddhism. Medical section of the *Mahavagga* (3rd section of the *Vinaya Piṭaka*) lists several therapeutic techniques like causing virility, curing impotence, giving emetics, purges of the upper and lower part of the body and of the head (*Śirōvirecana*), applying collyria (*anjana*), and ointments; ophthalmology, major surgery, pediatrics, giving of root medicines etc. All these techniques, described in *Mahavagga* are integral part of ayurveda. Medical service by the monks was freely available, because Buddhism does not permit payments in any kind. Buddhism inspired the idea of free medical services to all.

Many of the compositions that narrate the influence of Buddhism on ayurveda unequivocally refer to many situations when the disciples of Buddha have turned themselves to Buddha himself and requested solutions in medical problems.

Responding to a question about the causation of diseases by a *sramana* Sivaka, Gautama Buddha explained that the cause of the humankind's suffering (from diseases) is eightfold. 'bile (*pitta*), phlegm (*semha*), wind (*vāta*), and their combinations (*sannipata*), changes of the seasons (*utu*), stress of unusual activities (*viṣamaparihāra*) sitting or standing too long, going out hastily at night, and the result of (previous) actions (*kammavipāka*) is the eighth.

Here are some quotes from *Mahavagga* regarding medicine and its practice as suggested by Buddha; from *Buddhist Monastic Code* by Thanissaro Bhikku.

The Buddha sets out precise duties both for the sick and for those who nurse them: 'If one's preceptor is present, the preceptor should tend to one as long as life lasts (or) should stay until one's recovery. If one's teacher is present, the teacher should tend to one as long as life lasts (or) should stay until one's recovery. If one's pupil is present, the pupil should tend to one as long as life lasts (or) should stay until one's recovery….

'A sick person endowed with five qualities is easy to tend to: He does what is amenable to his cure; he knows the proper amount in things amenable to his cure; he takes his medicine; he tells his symptoms, as they actually are present, to the nurse desiring his welfare, saying that they are getting worse when they are getting worse, improving when they are improving, or remaining the same when they are remaining the same; and he is the type who can endure bodily feelings that are painful, fierce, sharp, wracking, repellent, disagreeable, life-threatening. A sick person endowed with these five qualities is easy to tend to.

'A nurse endowed with five qualities is not fit to tend to the sick: He is not competent at mixing medicine; he does not know what is amenable or unamenable to the patient's cure, bringing to the patient things that are unamenable and taking away things that are amenable; he is motivated by material gain, not by thoughts of good will; he gets disgusted at cleaning up excrement, urine, saliva, or vomit; and he is not competent at instructing, urging, rousing, and encouraging the sick person at the proper occasions with a talk on *dhamma*. A nurse endowed with these five qualities is not fit to tend to the sick.

'A nurse endowed with five qualities is fit to tend to the sick: He is competent at mixing medicine; he knows what is amenable or unamenable to the patient's cure, taking away things that are unamenable and bringing things that are amenable; he is motivated by thoughts of good will, not by material gain; he does not get disgusted at cleaning up excrement, urine, saliva, or vomit; and he is competent at instructing, urging, rousing, and encouraging the sick person at the proper occasions with a talk on *dhamma*. A nurse endowed with these five qualities is fit to tend to the sick.'

(Mahāvagga.VIII.26.1-8)

Buddhist literature mentions several herbs used in the preparation of medicines. They includeturmeric, ginger, sweet flag, white orris root, atis root, black hellebore, nut-grass, neem tree, kutaja (Wrightia antidysenterica), nattamala (Pongamia glabra) cucumber, cotton tree, vidanga (Embelia ribes), long pepper, black pepper, yellow myrobalan (Terminalia chebula), beleric myrobalan (Terminalia bellerica), emblic myrobalan (Phyllanthus embelica), asafoetida resin and mineral substances like sea salt, black salt, rock salt, culinary salt, red salt. They are classified intoseveral categories like root medicines, leaf medicines, fruit medicines etc.

These scriptures carried this knowledge to other parts of Asia too. Some important treatments for eye diseases, jaundice, wind afflictions etc. were mentioned in the literature.

For wind afflictions in the limbs: Sweating treatments, sweating treatments with herbs, and a 'great sweating' treatment are allowed. Use a hole dug lengthwise the size of a human being and fill it with burning embers, charcoal, or coals; cover it with sand or dirt, and then with various leaves that are good for wind diseases. Have the ill *bhikkhu* cover his body with oil and lie down on top of the leaves, turning over as necessary. Other treatments for wind afflictions in the limbs include hemp water (water boiled with hemp leaves) and a water tub, which is a tub big enough for a *bhikkhu* to get into. For wind affliction in the joints: Blood-letting and moxibustion are allowed.

For boils: Lancing (surgery) is allowed unless the boil is on the genitals or near the anus. Allowable post-operative treatments include astringent water, pounded sesame paste, a compress, and a bandage. The scar may be sprinkled with mustard-seed powder to prevent itching. It may also be fumigated, and the scar-tissue cut off with a piece of salt-crystal. The scar may also be treated with oil. An old piece of cloth is allowed for soaking up the oil, and every kind of treatment for sores or wounds is allowed.

For jaundice: Urine and yellow myrobalan are allowed. For a body full of bad humors: One may drink a purgative. After the purgative has worked, one may take clarified *conjee*, clear green gram broth, slightly thick green gram broth, or meat broth (broth without any meat).

Medical procedures: A *bhikkhu* who has surgery (lancing) or hemorrhoid removal performed in the crotch or within the area two fingerbreadths around it incurs a *thullaccaya*. Akasagotta shows the bikku, who has undergone the surgery to Buddha. The bhikku is not recovering. Buddha says 'how can this worthless man have surgery done in the crotch? In the crotch the skin is tender, a wound is hard to heal, the knife hard to guide.' Buddha has banished cruel surgeries that endanger the life of the patients. Mahavagga 6th chapter mentions several such treatments and nursing techniques.

The Pali term translated here as hemorrhoid removal *vatthi-kamma* (Skt. *vasti-karman*) usually translated as the administration of an enema. The idea of administering medicines through the anus may have first developed in the context of hemorrhoid treatment. The commentary adds that even trying to remove a hemorrhoid by squeezing it with a piece of hide or cloth would come under this prohibition. However, it recommends as a safer alternative that one apply an astringent decoction to the hemorrhoid and tie off the end with string. If the hemorrhoid then falls off on its own, well and good. Bloodletting is allowed as a treatment for wind afflictions of the joints.

Bhessajjakkandhaka (chapter on medicines) of the *Mahavagga* specifies the requisite medicines, namely, clarified butter (*sappi*), fresh butter (*navanīa*), oil (*tela*), honey (*madhu*), and molasses (*phanita*). With the evolution of *sangha* and the development of the *vinaya* rules, the medicines grew into an entire pharmacopoeia, which included *eranda* (Recinus communis), roots of turmeric (*haridra*), ginger (*Sṃgavera*), sweetflag (*vaca*), Indian atees (*ativiṣa*), black hellebore (*kaṭukarōhiṇi*), vetiver (*uśīra*), nut grass (*bhadramusta*), extracts of neem (*nimba* or Indian lilac), kurchi tree (*kuṭaja*), leaves of *nimba, kuṭaja,* snake gourd (*paṭōla*), holy basil (*tulasi*), cotton tree (*kārpāsa*), fruits of embelia (*viḍanga*), long pepper (*pippali*), pepper (*marīca*), yellow myrobalan (*haritaki*), beleric myrobalan (*vibhitaki*), emblic myrobalan (*āmalaki*), gums or resins of asafoetida (*hingu*), *lāksha*(lac), and salts like sea salt and rock salt. All these herbs and minerals must have been available with the physicians at the Buddhist monasteries. The range of medicines must be fairly large. The peppers and long peppers were traded from the ports of Malabar to Sindh and then on the land to north India. The material available in the Buddhist literature about medicine is spread across several parts. The knowledge is mostly practical and pragmatic. It aimed at results. Removing pain and consoling patient have been the chief aims of the vaidya. All these therapies described in the Buddhist literature are prominently discussed in ayurveda. Ayurveda boasts of alkali thread technique to heal hemorrhoids, *vastikarma* (enema), bloodletting etc all perfected during the Buddhist era.

Ayurveda looks at three causative factors of the diseases *viz.. indriya indriyārtha sannikarṣa* (interaction of sensory organs with the sensory stimuli), *prajnāparādha* (fallacy) and *pariṇāma* (seasonal changes). Buddha too emphasizes these causes as causative factors of all diseases. Caraka elaborates the concept of *karma*. This concept too, with certain different interpretations, is found in the theory of Buddhism. The meaning of *karma* varies between Buddhist outlook and that of Brahmanism.

Buddhism speculates that four subtle principles (*mahabhuta*) form the universe, *viz.. prithvi, ap, teja* and *vāyu*. Ayurveda treatises add *ākāṣa bhuta* (space) to them.

Buddhism was instrumental in shaping theory and practice of ayurveda and bringing the institutionalized medicine to India. Establishment of hospitals, hospices and old-age homes by the wandering mendicants and ascetics has necessitated the codification of medical knowledge. The ascetics also learnt the medicine to preach religion. Therefore, it was Buddhism that systematized ayurveda.

Nagarjuna

The problem of Nagarjuna is difficult to solve basing on the literary evidences, because in the history of India we find several persons with this name. There is a Buddhist Nagarjuna, ayurveda Nagarjuna, *rasāyana* (metallurgist) Nagarjuna, and a surgeon Nagarjuna. In Pataliputra (Patna in Bihar), an inscription mentions a formulation of Nagarjuna to treat conjunctivitis (acute viral inflammation of the eye). A surgeon Nagarjuna has rendered *uttara tantra* to *Suśrutasamhita*. Al-Biruni, who lived in India between the years 1017 and 1030 AD, alludes to Nagarjuna as an ayurveda physician belonging to fort Dihak near Somnath, a century ahead of him. One more Nagarjuna is linked to a village Vedali in the valley of the river Krishna in south India close to the Nagarjunakonda. This Buddhist Nagarjuna is probably residing in the valley of Srīparvata in Āndhradeśa.

The Tibetan sources ratify Nagarjuna born into an Andhra Brahmin family in the village of Vedali east to Sriparvata. He studied the *Veda*s and *Vādānga*s. From there he traveled to Pataliputra to worship goddess Sarasvati. At the age of eighteen, he became a Buddhist and began an in-depth study of ayurveda and Buddhist Philosophy. Kumarajiva's (AD 344) *Life of Bodhisatva Nagarjuna* says much about this young scholar. Kumarajiva went to China and translated many (Buddhist) Sanskrit works into Chinese. The Tibetan sources boast that Nagarjuna has lived for 500 years. Obviously, this indicates that several Nagarjunas lived in different times. The first Nagarjuna belonging to the 1st - 2nd centuries AD must be Bodhisatva Nagarjuna and later Nagarjuna an ayurvedic and alchemist Nagarjuna.

Ayurvedic medicine prior to (2nd) Nagarjuna comprised of preparations largely from vegetable sources. Nagarjuna founded *ras cikitsa* or *rasayan*, which was vehemently opposed by orthodox *vaidyas*. The *rasavaidyas* (medicinal alchemists), however, argue that the advantage of *rasa* is 'small dose and quick action', which protected the patient from consuming bitter concoctions. It is also argued that vegetable-based medicine becomes stale in the course of time while medicines comprising chemicals do not. The people too longed for quick and magic therapies instead of prolonged treatment with restricted diet.

The processes of 'distillation' and 'calcinations' are ascribed to Nagarjuna. According Cakradatta, the 12th century commentator of the *Carakasamhita,* Nagarjuna discovered *kajjavali*, the black sulphide of antimony. He was able to convert most metals into ashes/cinders and use them as medicines. Like modern chemotherapy, *rasāyana* medicine is efficient but can sometimes potentially harmful. The preparation of ashes (*bhasma*) is a tedious process and many mercurial preparations entail one thousand calcinations (*sahasrapuṭi*). Nagarjuna probably introduced mercury into India from Tibet during the Gupta kingdom. This period is known as *golden age* in Indian history. Mercury is not native to India and ayurveda. It is brought into India from China via Tibet and Kashmir. The Sanskrit word *pārada* indicates the name of the source, perhaps Pamir mountain range northwest of Indus. The Caraka and Suśruta are unaware of mercury. In the south perhaps, the Roman trade has introduced it into southern traditions.

Vagbhata in his *Aṣṭāngahṛdaya* lists the names of 27 *rasa siddha ācārya*s (erudite scholars in alchemy) and Nagarjuna is one of them. In spite of the nebulous historical facts around Nagarjuna, his or their contributions were watersheds in the history of ayurveda.

Ayurveda and Jainism

The world has reaped three influential religions, Judaism, Christianity and Islam in the Fertile Crescent of the Middle East. The Ganges civilization has offered other three great religions, Brahmanism, Jainism and Buddhism, to the world. The influence of Brahmanism is more on ayurveda from the Gupta period, 1500 years ago. However, the influence of Jainism and Buddhism on the efflorescence of ayurveda was much more than we think.

Prior to Buddhism, Jainism was the dominant faith in India. By the time of Buddha, Jainism was already a popular faith in the subcontinent. It preached extreme forms of compassion and non-violence often leading to self-punishments. Jainism had twenty-four *tirthankaras* or gurus in succession. The word *tirthankara* literally means ‘ford maker’, i.e. a person who builds bridge to cross the river. Jainism shows the way to *kaivalya*, emancipation. The founder of this faith was Rishabhanatha, also known as Adinatha. Historians conjuncture that this faith is as old as Indus civilization and more ancient than Brahmanism itself. The picture of ox (*ṛshabha*) in the Indus seals may be indicating the founder of Jainism. The 24th *tirthankara*, Mahavira was contemporary to Goutama Buddha. The 23rd *tirthankara*, Parsvanatha was probably the founder of core of this philosophy. He belonged to 8th century BC and lived in Kasi. Both Jain and Buddhist founders were born into *kṣatriya* (warrior) families. It is an important aspect in the history of India that the two great social reformers are not Brahmins. Therefore, they fought against caste system.

Jainism too has its immense influence on medicine. Like Brahmanism and Buddhism, Jainism originated in north India and spread to the south. Buddhism and Jainism rather competed in convincing the people about 'middle path' and extreme asceticism respectively. There are tens of

Jain religious sites in the north and south. A severe famine caused Jain believers to reach Karnataka during the days of Emperor Chandragupta Maurya along with Bhadrabahu, the distinguished leader of Jains. Thus, the Jain history in the South commences from the 3rd century B.C. Ācārya Bhadrabahu passed away in 297 B.C. at Shravanabelagola in Karnataka. Jainism continued as a popular faith for more than one thousand years in the peninsular India. Kondakundapuram (Konakondla) and Rayadurga (neighboring *Siddulakonda*) in Anantapur district of Andhra Pradesh have yielded rich archaeological data pointing to these sites as Jain educational centers.

Several kingdoms patronized Jainism. It is more respected in Karnataka and Rajasthan regions. Kadamba rulers (3rd – 6th c. AD), Ganga rulers (4th - 10th c. AD), Calukya rulers (6th – 8th c. AD), Rashtrakuta rulers (8th – 10th c. AD), Hoysala rulers (11th c. – 14th c. AD) in the south have patronized Jainism. The early Kākatiyas of Āndhradeśa too were Jains. The Vijayanagara Empire from 14th to 16th century has many Jain monks as ministers for kings.

Jains looked at the disease with real compassion. Jains discouraged primitive surgical techniques because such techniques cause immense pain in the subjects. Although ayurveda does not discriminate between the vegetarian and non-vegetarian sources of the food and medicine, Jainism propagated vegetarianism because of their loyalty to *ahimsa*, non-violence. Suicide is not pro-life and so ayurveda disapproves the act, while Jainism encourages it.

The Jains had a well-established tradition of medicine that was known as *prāṇavaya*. It deals with mental disciplines, dietetics and drugs and covers all the eight *angas* (branches) of ayurveda. It is the science of vitality to maintain healthy body and sane mind. The Jain saints looked after their health and their sickness themselves. They have forbidden alcohol, honey and meat and as a result, the Jain physicians had to modify the formulations accordingly because ayurveda extensively recommend them in the treatment. According to *Acarangasutra*, a Jain scripture, the 'nature' of plants and animals is similar. Plants and animals are living beings and so they too take birth, grow old, endure diseases and die. However, the Jains show more compassion toward the animals than the plants. Jains speculated about the birth of various living beings as can be seen from the examples given below:

From eggs (birds etc.)
From a foetus (elephant etc.)
From a foetus with an enveloping membrane (cow etc.)
From fluids (worms etc.)
From sweat (bugs etc.)
By coagulation (ants etc.)
From sprouts (butterflies etc.)
By regeneration (man etc.)

These ideas on birth of different life forms are also found in the literature of ayurveda. The *Cs, Ss* describe the genesis of life in their *śarirasthanas.*

The medicinal properties of mango, grapes, ginger, mustard stalks, *asvattha* (Ficus religiosa), *kadamba* (Anthocephalus cadamba), coconut, *kaseru* (Scirpus kysoor) lotus, sugarcane, *bilva* (Aegle marmelos) and garlic etc. are described. Cleanliness of body, speech and mind are important to stay healthy. Diabetes, anemia, epilepsy etc are described as very important diseases that affect the society.

The *Uttaradhyayana Sutra* is one of the most important sacred books of the Jains. It accepts sickness as one of the troubles. Different methods of treatment like spells, roots, emetics, purgatives, fumigation, anointing of the eye are discussed in detail. Use of inorganic substances such as metals, stones, mica, and sulfur are mentioned. However, the mercury is not mentioned.

Ugradityacharya authored *Kalyānakaraka* in 9th century AD. Interestingly, he mentioned the authors who had specialized in different branches of ayurveda.

Pujyapada – Śalākya (diseases of ear, nose, throat, teeth and eye)
Patrasvāmi – Śalya (general surgery)
Siddhasena – Visha and *graham (bhuta)* (toxicology and demonology)
Dasarathaguru – Kāyacikitsa (internal medicine)
Meghanada – Bālaroga (diseases of children)

Simhanāda – Rasāyana – Vājikaraṇa(gerontology and aphrodisialogy)

Samantabhadra – All the eight branches *(Aṣṭānga)*

The Jain tradition of medicine is often referred to as *Samantabhadra* school of medicine, as the sage Samantabhadra is dexterous in all eight branches of medicine. Actually, the South Indian tradition of ayurveda too is known as *samantabhadra* tradition; this shows the extent of Jain influence on medicine and society. The *Kalyānakaraka* is a good example to see the influence of religion on medicine. It avoids all animal products including ghee. The last three chapters of this treatise deal with surgical techniques, *pancakarma* and use of mercury along with its processing described respectively. The author says there is no penance greater than *cikitsa* (treatment). '*Cikitsa* is for destroying sins and promoting virtues'.

Jains considered disease as the result of sin. Therefore, they were passive recipients of medical treatment rather than active promoters of the same like Buddhists. They discouraged animal products in preparing medicines. Although ayurveda treatises carry ample number of medicinal preparations containing animal products, the Jaina influence has considerably reduced their number in treatment.

The *Saidapura* Inscription (1034 AD) in Nalgonda district of Telangana is in Sanskrit. It says, Aggalayya, a famous surgeon in the court of the king, undertakes difficult cases and helps the patients. For his services, Aggalayya was honored with a title *Naravaidya* (doctor of humans). He received titles *Pranācārya* (professor of life science) and *Vaidyaratnakara* (jewel among the doctors). Aggalayya professed Jainism. Aggalayya was a famous surgeon like Suśruta around that place. Aggalayya's life is an example to disprove that the Jainism has banished surgery in ayurveda. Until the invention of anesthesia in Europe in the

19th century, the surgery was painful and desisted by the patients. The treatment is worse than disease in the absence of anesthesia. Buddha has recommended certain guidelines to avoid pain during surgery. Jainism too condemned painful surgeries; however, Buddhism and Jainism have not barred the practice of surgery. In the later period, Jainism has lost ground to Śaivism in south India. Because of this, ayurveda has not retained the elements of Jainism i.e. prohibition of animal-derived products in medicine.

Surgery in Ancient India

An emphasis on surgery is found in the *Suśrutasamhita.* Often Suśruta was projected by the historians of ayurveda as the first surgeon in the world. Complex surgeries were indeed described in the *Suśrutasamhita* in situations like difficult childbirth, urinary crystals obstructing urination, repairing noses, extracting lumps etc. The patients had to be congratulated, rather than surgeons, for undergoing and tolerating such surgeries in the days of absence of anesthesia. The skill of the ancient surgeons was certainly comparable to the modern surgeons but lack of knowledge of fine anatomy was challenging. Bleeding and shock were two problems that could not be surpassed by the ancient surgeons. Post-operative care was another difficult task.

The ayurvedic word for surgery is *śalya*, a foreign body lodged in the human body. Many diseases described in *śalākya*, the supra-clavicular diseases (diseases of Ear, Nose, Throat, Eyes) are treated medically. Surgeons of those days were mostly well versed in extracting arrowheads, thorns from the soles, lancing the boils, fixing the fractures etc. The treatises described One hundred and twenty one surgical instruments, (101 blunt and 20 sharp). One hundred and one blunt instruments were grouped into six categories: twenty four *svastikayantra* (scissors like), *samdamsa yantra* (forceps like), some are like tubes and some are like spoons. Suśruta lauds the hand as the most important instrument!

Suśruta described the basic surgical techniques in eight categories. They are *chedana* (cutting), *bhedana* (incision), *lekhana* (scrapping), *vyadhana* (making holes), *eṣana* (exploring/probing), *aharana* (extracting), *visrāvana* (ooze out), *sivana* (suturing). Instruments were heated on fire to prevent the post-operative complications. Catheterization (inserting a tube into the urinary bladder to facilitate urinations), using leaches for bloodletting, cautery were also in practice.

Rhinoplasty is a well-known technique of reconstruction of nose, an original invention of Indian surgeons. Indian society used to punish criminals by severing nose and ears. Those unfortunates consulted the surgeons, who creatively incise and fold down the skin of the cheek on the place of nose to rebuild it. In the middle ages, this caste skill has stimulated the plastic surgery in Europe. The *Suśrutasamhita* describes piercing of the ear, correcting repairing split ear lobes, bloodletting and other surgeries.

Couching, a technique of cataract surgery

was described by Suśruta. In this technique, the surgeon dislodges the opaque lenses of the eye. This technique is no longer considered scientific by the ophthalmologists. This technique was mentioned in the Hammurabi code (18th c. B.C.) too in Babylonia and it was a widespread practice across the world. In essence, the surgery described and practiced in ancient India is just history of modern surgery and it cannot claim a special status, as expected by the ayurveda surgeons.

Ayurveda beyond the subcontinent

In *Carakasamhita* and *Suśrutasamhita*, we read at several places about the students coming to India to study ayurveda. Bahlika, Gandhara, and many such names of foreign places appear in the treatises. It was due of Buddhist monks; the word of ayurveda has spread to other regions in Asia. This process has augmented integration of Asian medical systems. There are innumerable parallels between the concepts of ayurveda and traditional systems of other civilizations of Greece, Egypt, Mesopotamia and China. Vigorous exchanges of information certainly happened between these civilizations. The trade and migrations facilitated this transmission. Moreover, the subcontinent has favorable location between the east and the west.

The coast of peninsular India has unique seasonal drifts of the seawater. During the southwest monsoon, the seawater drifts from the west to the east, circling the Indian peninsula and in the winter from the east to the west, i.e. in the opposite direction. The sea and ocean currents elsewhere on the globe have fixed perennial patterns. They do not change their course of direction. However, there is one exception. The south-west monsoon-drift (warm ocean current that flows on the surface of the Arabian Sea) from the East Africa towards India and beyond, is active in the summer. This current pushes the ships along the coast of Asia. After six months, this current reverses during the Northeast monsoon. These seasonal variations helped the Indian traders to transport goods between nations. The peninsular part of south India has lengthy coastline along the Arabian Sea in the west and the Bay of Bengal in the east. The Arabian Sea and the Bay of Bengal are two arms of the Indian Ocean. The tradesmen ventured to the eastern lands (Malaya, Java and Sumatra) in the summer and returned in the winter. Some tradesmen from south ventured to the western lands (Arabia) in winter and returned in the summers.

Traders from Roman Empire and the Middle East could trade with the south India depending on these sea drifts augmented by the Trade Winds. This interaction (the Middle East and Europe with South India) has also influenced the growth of traditional medicine. The trade between the west and South India is proved by the hoards of Roman coins from Tamilnadu and Andhra Pradesh. The list of traded items is very long. Spices always topped the list. Edward Gibbon in his historical *Decline and Fall of Roman Empire* acknowledges the trade with India '.....the ambassadors expressed their gratitude to the bounteous lady of the village, by a very acceptable present of silver cups, red fleeces, dried fruits, and Indian pepper..'

The warm-water surface drifts of the Indian

Ocean helped Indian merchants to import and export grains, herbs and other merchandise with the countries in east and west. Marco Polo, Vasco-da-Gama and many other visitors have reached the coast of India using these sea-drifts caused by periodical winds and the rotation of the earth. During the Cola period from 10th century AD, ayurveda spread to South East Asian nations from the Indian peninsula. Rich cultural and architectural heritage in South East Asia proves the fact that ayurveda sailed across the Bay of Bengal and got popularized in Suvarnadvipa (Indonesia), Kambhoja (Cambodia), Campa (Vietnam). By the end of 10th century AD, Buddhism lost its hold on the society. The universities that once attracted students from neighboring countries gradually declined. Śaivism and Brahmanism dominated the society. The verve that once energized the scholars of ayurveda started disappearing. Gradually a state of stagnation ruled over ayurveda. The stratified society was not allowed to integrate itself. The caste was the prime culprit for this stagnation in the society. For the people of India caste is the religion!

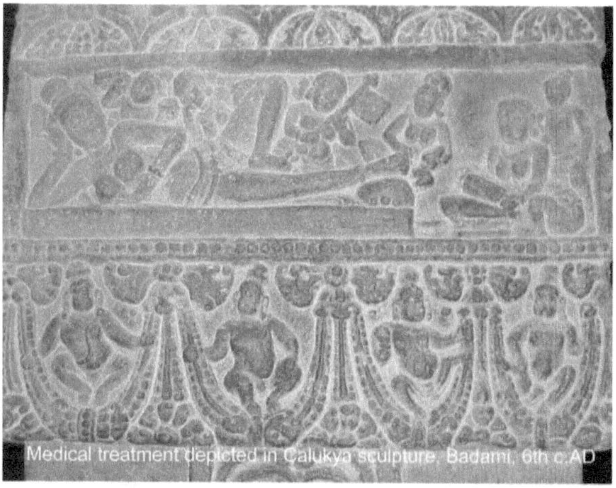
Medical treatment depicted in Calukya sculpture, Badami, 6th c.AD

A nursing scenario from 6th c. AD

Chapter Three

AYURVEDA IN THE MEDIEVAL PERIOD

God heals and the Doctor takes the fee.
- Benjamin Franklin, (1706-1790)

Historians consider the medieval period of Europe beginning in the 5thcentury AD, after the collapse of Western Roman Empire, and ending with the commencement of Renaissance and the Age of Discovery in the 15th century AD. The European historians and historians of India tried to classify the history of India into classical, medieval and modern periods. From the point of view of political history of India, the medieval period has not commenced immediately after the fall of Gupta Empire in the 6th century AD. The King Harsha continued the legacy of political achievements, practice religious tolerance, patronized Buddhism and literature until his death in 647 AD. In the south, the Calukya king Pulakesti II forced Harsha to limit his kingdom only up to the river Narmada in central India. India was ruled by benevolent rulers up to the 7th century AD in the north. The south India has never yielded to Islamic invasions until the process of colonization has started by the European powers. Therefore, medieval period of ayurveda does not synchronize with the political events.

After the appearance of the *Mādhavanidāna* in the 8th century AD, the literature of ayurveda has experienced a state of stagnation. This period coincides with the Islamic invasion of north India. The heartland of north India has come under Islamic ruling from 10th century AD onwards. It took almost five centuries for the Islamic forces to quash big Hindu kingdoms of the south and east. The Ganga dynasty of Orissa started declining in the 15th c. AD. The early medieval period of India, therefore, started in the 9th century AD and continued until the establishment of Moghul period in the 16th century AD. The late medieval period lasted until the dissolution of the Moghul Empire. During the medieval period, several kingdoms ruled different regions of the subcontinent. The Cola Empire in the south was at its height from 9th to 13th centuries; Hoysala Empire in Karnataka region between 10th and 14th centuries, Kakatiya kingdom in Andhra region between 11th to 14th centuries and Vijayanagar Empire ruled almost entire south India from 14th century till 16th century AD.

Between the 10th and 15th centuries, AD ayurveda had a new companion, yunani medicine. Strengthened by the wisdom and medical philosophies of the Middle East, yunani medicine was patronized by the Muslim rulers. Surprisingly, the diagnostics, pharmacopoeia and therapeutics of yunani and ayurveda are analogous to each other. The main reason for similarities between the yunani and ayurveda is not just the coexistence for millennia but also their common roots prior to the Indus civilization. Ayurveda physicians of the medieval period have produced voluminous encyclopedias, thesauri and independent treatises on ayurveda. The two of the so-called lesser triad (*laghutrayi*), *Bhāvaprakāśa* and *Śārangadhara samhita* appeared during this period. The *Mādhavanidāna* had appeared little earlier.

Ayurveda during the Vijayanagara Period

The Vijayanagara Empire was founded in 1336 AD by Harihara I and his brother Bukka I with Hampi (Vijayanagara) as capital city on the southern bank of river Tungabhadra, a tributary to the river Krishna in south India. It arrested the expansion of the Muslim power for more than two centuries. Although it lasted until 1646 AD, its sphere of power waned after the defeat at Tallikota war in 1565 AD. The combined army of the South sultanates of the Deccan (Bijapur, Golconda, Ahmednagar, Bahmani) has ravaged the city's splendor and it could never recover. Vijayanagara, the City of Victory, was a proud city of South India. The writings of medieval European travelers such as Domingo Paes, Fernao Nuniz and Niccolò Da Conti, literature in Telugu and Kannada languages and the archaeological excavations at Hampi provide crucial information about this empire. Substantial portion of south India came under the sway of Vijayanagara. Two hundred and thirty years of stable empire and royal patronage were congenial to growth of ayurveda.

Efficient administration and vigorous overseas trade brought new technologies like water management systems for irrigation boosting the population. Several *vaidyas* have compiled ayurvedic texts. Innumerable new herbs found their way into the pharmacopoeia of ayurveda. Some important treatises of ayurveda namely the *Basavarājīya*, the *Vaidyarājavallabha*, the *Vaidyacintāmani* and the *Bahāṭam* were compiled during this period.

Lakshmana Pandita or Lakshmanācārya served Immadi Bukka as physician and authored *Vaidyarājavallabha*, also known as *Vallabharājīya*. In the introductory chapter of *Vaidyarājavallabha*, Laxmana Pandita eulogized the valor and victories of Immadi Bukka, the ruler of Hampi. With the Vijayanagara Kingdom now imperial in stature, Harihara II, the second son of Bukka Raya I, further consolidated the kingdom beyond the river Krishna and brought the whole of South India under the Vijayanagara umbrella. Vishnusarma, an Ayurveda scholar had served under Harihara II of Vijayanagara Empire in the 14th century AD. In the vast expanse of ruins of the capital city of Hampi, the palace of Vira Harihara, who ruled the Vijayanagara Empire from 1377 to 1404, was located. In the palace premises, the bathroom and toilet too were identified. The toilet is linked to an underground pit lined by stones on the sides.

After nearly two decades of conflict with rebellious chieftains, the empire eventually came under the rule of Krishnadevaraya, the son of Tuluva Narasa Nayaka. Acclaimed as one of the greatest in Indian history, Krishnadevaraya (1509 to 1529 AD) became synonymous with military glory, economic prosperity, good administration, and artistic splendor. During this period, Telugu and Kannada literature flourished as never before. He himself has authored the *Amuktamalyada* (unworn garland's), which describes ayurveda in more than one place. Srikrishnadevaraya opines that the doctors have to be paid less money because more money easily corrupts them. Srikrishnadevaraya is known for his strict daily regimen according to the principles of ayurveda as described by Domingo Peas, a contemporary Portuguese visitor.

The excavations at Vijayanagara brought to light the remains of a well-connected water distribution system existing solely within the royal enclosure and the large temple complexes. The Noble men's quarters have shown that each house has a private well and conduits to carry bathroom water out. Near the *mahānavami dibba* (*dasara dibba*), a beautiful stone platform, public urinals were identified. A long stone water tank is seen near the king's assembly, used for horses to drink water. The *dasaradibba*, the victory podium amid the ruins of Hampi show delicately carved out images on stone depicting the tradesmen from Persia parading before the kings with their merchandise that includes beautiful women from Persia.

The empire's economy was largely dependent on agriculture. Corn (*jowar*), cotton and pulse legumes grew in semi arid regions, while sugarcane, rice and wheat thrived as wet crops. Betel leaves, areca nut and coconut were the principal cash crops. Spices such as turmeric, pepper, cardamom and ginger grew in the remote Malnad hill region and were transported to the city for trade. Betel leaf was a favorite pastime of the people. Domingo Peas reports that 'betel is an herb which has a leaf like the leaf of the pepper, or the ivy of our country; they always eat this leaf, and carry it in their mouths with another fruit called areca. This is something like a medlar, but it is very hard, and it is very good for the breath and has many other virtues; it is the best provision for those who do not eat as we do. Some of them eat flesh;

they eat all kinds except beef and pork, and yet, nevertheless, they cease not to eat this betel all day'. The betel leaf, areca nut and turmeric have assumed greater cultural significance in India. Exchanging of betel leaf indicates an auspicious social agreement.

The main imports on the east coast were non-ferrous metals, camphor, porcelain, silk and luxury goods. The narrative of Duarte Barbosa, a cousin of Magellan, who visited the Vijayanagara city between 1504 AD and 1514 AD, describes large trade of the seaport of Bhatkal on its western coast, the exports from which consisted of iron, spices, drugs, myrobalans, and the imports of horses and pearls. Myrobalans are known as *triphala*, three fruits. *Triphala* is the prime medicine in ayurveda. Myrobalans also figure in the list of traded goods between India and England during the colonial period. The Terminalia chebula, *harītaki*, was used in medicine, tanning of leather and preparing ink.

Around one million people inhabited the city of Vijayanagara. Robert Sewell in his epoch-making book, the *Forgotten Empire*, has touched upon various public constructions like temples and other structures with an idea of hygiene. Now dilapidated Krishna temple in Hampi has a huge water tank hewn out of a single granite stone with opening to take water by the visiting devotees. Suravaram Prathapa Reddy in his *Andhrula Sānghika Caritra* (Social history of Andhras) alludes to an ayurveda school in Hampi during the 14th and 15th centuries AD, which was frequented by the students from abroad as well. This description was based on travelogues of Sulaiman and Fluger. A city with one million populations must have been a haven for ayurveda physicians and so there must be a school for them. Archaeological evidence is yet to emerge from ongoing excavations.

Contemporary to Vijayanagara Empire, there flourished Islamic kingdoms north to Hampi. The yunani as well as ayurveda flourished in those kingdoms. The life of the physicians was not easy in the middle ages. Physicians are acclaimed in the peacetime and the better services are demanded at critical times. When physicians fail in saving lives they were even executed by the rulers. Sultan Ibrahim of Bijapur was in the death bed in the year 1557 AD. During his illness, he put to death several physicians who had failed to cure him, beheading some, and causing others to be trodden to death by elephants, so that all the surviving medical practitioners, alarmed, fled from his dominions. We don't find the instances of such punishments being awarded to the ayurveda physicians in the ayurveda literature.

The popularity of ayurveda was more among the elite sections of the society than among the rural population until the end of 17th century AD. Majority of the population depended on home remedies and expertise of the grandmother or local physicians whose medical knowledge was limited but appropriate to the local needs. Ayurveda, like any other occupation, is inherited in some families as a profession, who mostly served with the local feudal lords and kings.

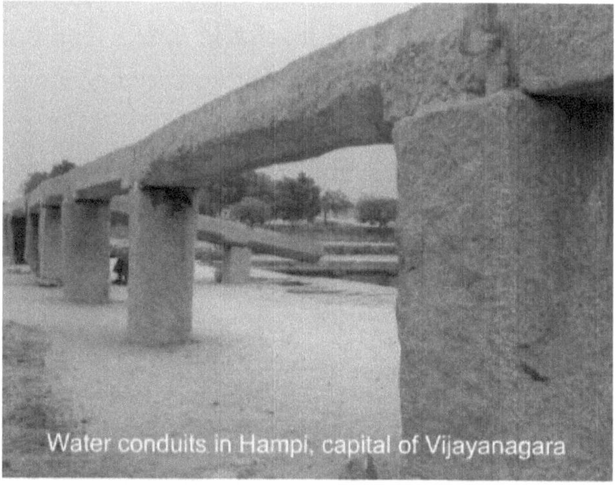
Water conduits in Hampi, capital of Vijayanagara

Diagnostics

Aṣṭasthāna parīkṣa (eightfold examination) is a method of testing *jihva* (tongue), *netra* (eyes), *nāḍi* (pulse), *mutra* (urine), *mala* (feces), *śabda* (voice), *sparśa* (touch) and *rupa* (appearance) in diagnosis. The *Yogaratnākara* of the late 17th century has detailed this method of examination. The testing of these eight parameters is useful to assess the state of disease causing humors. Certainly, this method came into popularity in India in medieval period.

It is surprising not to find any explanation of pulse (*nāḍi*) in the *Caraka* and *Suśrutasamhitas*. The pulse-lore, the knowledge of pulse in diagnosis, plays a pivotal role in Chinese, siddha and yunani medicines. The *Śārangadharasamhita*, of the 13th century AD narrates technique of pulse observation for the first time in India. The *Yōgaratnakara* of

Nayanasekhara deals with *nāḍi* in detail. The pulse helps physician to assess predominance of humor(s).

The *Caraka* and *Suśrutasamhitas* do not depend on pulse to estimate the vitiation of humors. In siddha too, the examination of pulse appears to be of recent origin. Siddha literature refers to a siddhar, Bogor, who reportedly visited China during the Cola period and brought it to Dravidadeśa. Medical historians consider him as a contemporary to the king Rajaraja in 9th century AD.

The pulse examination is very ancient in Persian and Arab civilizations and so this is not new to yunani medicine. It is also possible that the yunani medicine has contributed this concept to ayurveda in the north. The available data is inconclusive to point to the exact period or person, from north or south, who introduced it to ayurveda. Most probably, as the *Aṣṭasthānaparīkṣa* is central in diagnostics, the pulse-lore too has spread from the Dravidadeśa.

Ayurveda was never a static subject. It constantly accepted new concepts and practices into its fold. Using old words for new concepts is common in every culture. *Nāḍi* is pulsating radial artery. The artery is a vessel that carries oxygenated blood to the tissues. The veins carry the de-oxygenated blood back to the heart. The capillaries link the arteries and veins. Arteries run deep while the veins criss-cross under the surface of the skin. In some places, arteries flow near the surface, e.g. radial artery. It is felt just below the thumb on the wrist. It reflects flow, volume and pressure of the blood. Measuring pulse rate is not important in any traditional medicine because the chronometer was not available then. Instead, its *behavior* is examined. Ayurveda physicians consider arteries and veins as dhamani and sira. However, ayurveda *samhitas* do not distinguish them in such a way. The word *nāḍi* was used to denote nerve by today's ayurveda vocabulary. Therefore, the word chosen for pulse indicates that the practice of pulse examination is not indigenous. If pulse examination is indigenous to ayurveda, the word *dhamani* was to be chosen. Apparently, the practice of pulse examination is adopted from either siddha medicine or yunani medicine. The *Suśrutasamhita* proves beyond dispute that the ancient ayurvedists have conducted dissections on the dead body to understand and appreciate the internal structure of the human body. When the cadaver is opened, the arteries appear as empty tubes due to high elasticity of the arterial walls. Therefore, the blood is ejected into veins. Veins bulge with blood and arteries appear empty in a dead body. The nerves appear white and tube like. Therefore, ayurvedists mistook the arteries as wind-carrying pipes linked to the breathing apparatus. This comprehension on internal tubular structures could not have allowed ayurveda physicians to independently discover the pulse as a useful diagnostic tool.

Some important contents of the *Aṣṭasthānaparikṣa* like *mala* (feces) and *mutra* (urine) *parīkṣa* too were adopted from yunani medicine. The purpose of these examinations is to assess the state of the humors in the body. The examination of the urine is prognostic rather than diagnostic. The type of spread of an oil drop on the surface of urine is interpreted to forecast recovery or doom.

Some important treatises

Though there is no headway in medical science, several treatises were authored by the scholars of ayurveda. Many of these treatises were mere repetitions sans new ideas. Often many scholars wrote books to appease the kings and local lords. However, many of those texts still are popular among the ayurveda physicians today.

After the 10th century A.D., ayurveda treatises were composed with an emphasis on para-clinical aspects, i.e. pharmacology, pathology etc. The *Mādhavanidāna* is considered to be the most authentic work on *nidāna* (pathology) vividly describing the signs and symptoms of common diseases. Authored by Madhavakara in 8th century A.D. this composition is venerated by all ayurveda physicians across India. It imported lot of material from earlier Big Three texts.

The *Śārangadhara samhita* was written by Śārangadhara in 13th century AD. This composition is an update of medicine. Today, many ayurvedic pharmacies follow the formulations from this treatise. Historians call him progressive thinker of the middle ages. Śārangadhara has proposed an idea of link between the respiration and digestive fire analogous to iron smith's furnace. Śārangadhara might have spent sleepless nights to understand the physiology behind respiration. His imagination remained a hypothesis. He thought the air that is breathed in reaches the stomach to invigorate the digestive fire. He also speculated on the human locomotion. Earlier, the scholars of ayurveda considered the muscles as 'fortifying' constituents of the body. Muscle tissue (*māmsadhātu*) is packed in the fibers of muscle (*peśi*) and its function is to cover the bones according to Suśruta. Śārangadhara opined that the muscles are responsible for the locomotion; a new idea at that point of time. He also added several exotic substances like mercury, opium and other material, which entered India, to the pharmacology of ayurveda.

The *Bhāvaprakāśa* was written by Bhavamisra of 16th century AD. Bhavamisra has described more than 500 vegetable and animal products used in ayurveda along with their identification and usage. The *Bhāvaprakāśa* was the first to describe the disease syphilis in ayurveda. The *Mādhavanidāna*, the *Bhāvaprakāśa* and the *Śārangadhara* are known as Lesser Three (*laghutrayi*).

Cārucarya (Worthy Regimen)

The *Cārucarya*, authored by the king Bhoja in later half of the 11th century AD, is an interesting semi-medical work that reflects the society of medieval India. This book is basically a treatise on social and preventive medicine and gives lots of hints on enjoying physical life. It tells how to distinguish between good and bad areca nuts, explains the differences among the qualities of saffron from Kashmir and Persian countries, classifies women into different categories and suggests that those who copulate with low-caste house cleaners will shorten their lifespan. The *Cārucarya* is an encyclopedic work on daily life. It emphasizes on good *dinacarya* (daily routine) to make life happier. Although it's a guide to good health, it reflects the lifestyle of the feudalistic society. The myths and superstitions that dominated the society at that time have crept into this work. *Cārucarya* helped the aristocratic section of the society to draw pleasures in life rather than with an aim of progress in medicine. This treatise does not deal with diseases and treatment.

Vaidya Cintāmani

This treatise is also known as *Andhra vaidya cintamani*. Indrakanti Vallabhācārya (14th -15th centuries AD), probably from coastal Āndhradeśa, compiled it. The *Basavarājīyam* has quoted extensively from this composition verbatim. An important feature of this composition is the description of *Aṣṭasthānaparīkṣa*, the examination of pulse, voice, tongue, body appearance, touch, urine and feces to diagnose diseases. Till the appearance of the *Basavarājīyam* a century later, this composition has commanded the respect of all Ayurveda physicians.

The new treatments found in this work are:

1. Vallabhācārya added new signs and symptoms of *mahajvara* (chronic fevers).

2. He added new category of *mahakhsaya* (serious or chronic tuberculosis) to *kṣaya* (tuberculosis) diseases.

3. He added new variants of *kāsa* (cough), *bangala kāsa* and *mandara kāsa*. The word *kāsa* indicates not merely cough but any respiratory disease with cough.

4. He recommended boiled urine, resin of *velaga* (wood apple) and *phiranga* (papaya) wood for treatment in diabetes.

5. He prescribed *postukaya* (poppy fruit), *gasagasalu* (seeds of Papaver somniferum) and *ahiphena* in stomach ulcers.

6. In the diseases of ano-rectal region he recommended *gauripashana* (Arsenic penta sulphide). *Gauripashana* is red in colour. The yellow variety of *gauripashana* is Arsenic tri-sulphide, commonly known as yellow orpiment.

7. He prescribed opium (*ahiphena*) in chronic gastro-enteritis.

8. In indigestion, he recommended the ash of seeds collected from *ummetta* (Datura stromonium).

9. In severe throat infections (*kanthajihvaka kasa*) with cough, he recommended smoking the roots of *nepala* (Baliospermum montanum).

10. He recommended mercury in *yuka* (lice in the hair).

Use of opium was popular in South India according to some prescriptions from this treatise. *Vaidyacintāmani* is hardly consulted by the ayurveda physicians these days and it is very difficult to see a printed copy of this book in the libraries of ayurveda colleges of India.

Basavarājīyam

Kotturu Basavaraja (15th - 16th centuries AD) belongs to an Andhra Brahmin family. The town Kottur is near the present day Hospet in Karnataka state. Basavaraja records at the end of every chapter about his place. He belongs to Nidimamidi village in Āndhradeśa. This village can be identified with Nidimamidi near Puttaparthy of Anantapur district in Andhra Pradesh. His ancestors had migrated from Kottur to Nidimamidi much earlier hence the surname Kotturu. He composed this work after consultation of standard ayurveda treatises like the *Caraka, Mādhavanidāna, Cintamani, Rasārnava* and quoted from them extensively. This composition is highly respected among the Telugu and Kannada *vaidyas*. Basavaraja revises some classical prescriptions and adds not-so-popular folk medicines into mainstream ayurveda. As quoted above he has extensively copied from the *Vaidyacintāmani*. Like any other ayurveda treatise, the *Basavarājīyam* begins with the chapter on *Jvara* (fever).

These are few samples from the treatise.
1. *Karpari* in chronic fevers. (Skt. *plakṣa*).
*Karpari*is the name given to Indian tulip tree and it also indicates a kind of river sediment.

2.*Vishamuṣṭi* (Strychnos nuxvomica) in

agnimāndya (indigestion)
3. *Balurakkasi* (Agave angustifolia) in *ubbasam* (asthma)
4. Gum from neem tree in diabetes.
5.*Navāsāram* (Salammoniac or Ammonium chloride) in *pratiśyāyam* (common cold).

Surprisingly in Europe too this was used as expectorant till better anti-tussives were discovered.
6. *Mayura tutta* (cupric sulphate) in *yonisula* (pain in vagina).
7. Dropping few drops of blood collected from an ear of pig in *unmāda* (insanity)
8. Seeds of *gunja* (Abrus precatorius) in heart diseases.

An important character of the *Basavarājīyam* is its belief in the *karmavipāka*. The 24th chapter exclusively deals with the diseases caused by sins against the society, Brahmins and the god. Diseases are caused, according to Basavaraja, by behaving against the prevailing moral code of the society.

Outside mainstream ayurveda, several self-trained physicians still follow this treatise. *Basavarājiyam* is not an important treatise forthe physicians today. Nonetheless, it is very popular in south India.

Yōgaratnākaram

It is one of the renowned treatises of ayurveda written in the 17th century. It fulfills the lacunae of the earlier ayurveda treatises by elaborating different chapters on diagnosis, formulation of medicines and range of herbal and mineral products. This work has risen to prominence in the 18th and 19th centuries, when ayurveda colleges were first established under the British in Mysore and Madras, the *Yogaratnākaram* was recommended as textbook of ayurveda. Profulla Chandra Roy in his *History of Hindu*

Chemistry opines that the *Yōgaratnākaram* was composed in the 16th century or even earlier.

The *Yōgaratnākaram* describes the examination of pulse (*nāḍi-parīkṣa*) as part of the eight-fold examination (*aṣṭasthāna-parīkṣa*). One of the meanings of 'yoga' is 'pharmaceutical preparation'. The *Yōgaratnākaram* deals with several ayurveda topics except *śarira racana* (anatomy) and *śalya cikitsa* (surgery). This treatise uses pulse examination for both diagnosis and prognosis. Cannabis indica (*ganja*) is extensively recommended in several preparations. A noteworthy observation in the *Yōgaratnākaram* is the description of tobacco. New beverages like *sara, panaka* were introduced by the *Yōgaratnākaram*. The popular and inevitable dish in everyday meal of South India, *caru*, is lauded in this work. This work is stated to have been composed by Nayana Sekhara but there is no conclusive evidence.

It talks about 4 varieties of mercury (*rasa*) and compares them to 4 *varnas* of the society. *sveta* (white), *rakta* (red), *pīta* (bluish) and *kriṣṇa* (black) *varnas* are ascribed to mercury depending on its purity. It treats herbal and mineral products with equal importance. Pulse examination is described in 48 verses and 33 variations of pulse behavior were observed by the author.

Viadyajivana

The *Vaidyajivana* (livelihood of a physician) is written by Lōlambarāja. Colin Mackenzie has catalogued it under Telugu language; however,

Lolambaraja is proved to be a scholar from Maratha region. The author describes the beauty of his wife along with ayurveda in this text.

Hundreds of manuscripts were collected pertaining to ayurveda scripted in the medieval period. Several manuscript libraries host these collected material. *Vaidyagrantha* is an incomplete text of an unknown author. It describes anatomy, treatment of the diseases of women and children, childbirth and several common diseases. It was written in Telugu. *Śaḍrasa Nighanṭu* is an exclusive work on pharmacology. *Chikitsa śataślōka* is a treatise on several common diseases with Telugu commentary. *Hara Pradipika* is an exclusive treatise on alchemy with Telugu commentary.

Nighanṭus

Nighanṭu is a sort of thesaurus. The emergence of these works started in the medieval ages, when the identification of the medicinal plants has become a specialized knowledge. They describe the morphology, synonyms and *rasa, guṇa, vīrya* and *vipāka* of the drugs. Some important *Nighanṭus* of ayurveda are *Dhanvantari Nighanṭu, Madanapala Nighanṭu, Kayyadeva Nighanṭu* and *Aṣṭānga Nighanṭu*.

The *Nighanṭus* occupy a special place in ayurveda. All these *Nighanṭus* classify edibles and drug substances into several categories. The purpose of the *Nighaṇṭu* is to help the medical students to memorize the names of the herbs and their application.The *Nighaṇṭus* were kept updated with the arrival of new herbs.

Majority of works that appeared in the middle ages were handbooks for the practicing physicians. The tradition of writing a *samhita*-kind of work has become outdated in the middle ages. The first such handbook of therapeutics *sidhayoga* was written by Vrinda in the 9th century AD. *Cakradatta,* another such handbook was compiled by Cakrapani in the 11th century AD.

Rasāyana and Alchemy

Alchemy is an Arabic word for chemistry. *Rasāyana*, as described in ayurveda treatises, is a branch of medicine to restore and prolong healthy living by using several herbs like *harītaki* (Terminalia chebula), *āmalaki* (Embilia officinalis) etc. This is equivalent to geriatrics, treating the diseases of the old age. Therefore, the word *rasa* does not indicate mercury in ancient Indian medicine. The words *Rasaśāstra* and *Rasatantra* are used to denote medicinal alchemy. The use of mercury is not found in the *Carakasamhta*, the *Suśrutasamhita* and the *Aṣṭāngahṛdaya samhita.* Use of mercury in medicine and claims of transmutation of mercury into gold are medieval in origin. All *rasaśāstra/rasatantra* compositions like *Rasaratna samuchchaya* (Pile of mercurial preparations), *Rasarnava* (Ocean of mercury),

Rasatarangini (Adobe of waves of mercury) belong to medieval period. Although mercury was available prior to medieval period, it took few centuries to develop a branch of medicinal alchemy revolving around mercury. Mercury was imported into India from Italy and China.

The word *rasa* has several meanings in ayurveda. *Rasa* = essence, juice, taste, mercury, gold, nourishing liquid, connoisseur and even semen of the god Siva. *Ayana* = way, path, realm. Mehdihassan, the author of a remarkable book *Indian Alchemy or Rasāyana*, takes the meaning of *ayana* etymologically. He translates the word *rasāyana* as 'path of mercury'. But *ayana* in Sanskrit denotes several shades of the similar meanings. For instance: *Rāmāyana* (the story of Rama, or Rama's journey) and *uttarayana* (sun's shift to north). Both may indicate path or journey but over the centuries, the word *ayana* has gathered new connotations. Therefore, the nearest meaning of *rasāyana* is 'realm of mercury'. *Rasatantra / Rasaśāstra* deal with the branch of preparation of medicines using herbo-minerals or purely mineral substances.

The yellow metal is admired for its enduring colour and brilliance. Using gold either in the form of metal or cinder in food and medicine was prevalent among the affluent section of the society. Man searched for ways to 'produce' gold because mining is cumbersome.Many kingdoms dreamed to discover Eldorado, the gold mine. The thirst for yellow metal led brave people to explore the world and experimentation in chemistry.

The reasons for the entry of mercury into ayurveda pharmacopoeia are very clear. Treating minerals with the herbs may impart the qualities of herbal growth into metals. Metals used in the form of medicines are believed to induce strength and durability into the body. Because the gold is valued as the supreme of all metals, implanting gold into the framework of human body is believed to be an important process to prolong life. The ancient physicians wanted to make human body invincible by administering gold in different forms.This hope and ample supply of mercury from the Roman Empire as well as China had stimulated the art of alchemy and *rasaśāstra* in South India. Several ayurveda physicians chose alchemy as their profession.

Alchemy was a worldwide phenomenon. Indian alchemy uses mercury, sulfur, gold, silver, tin, iron and other earthen material like mica to prepare medicines. Several herbs are employed to process the crude alloys and metals to instill certain characteristics of herbs into metals. Transmutation of lower metals into gold was a dream. Al-Biruni, a mathematician and astronomer from central Asia (Uzbekistan), who visited India in 11th century AD and studied Indian sciences, states that 'Indians have a science similar to the alchemy which is quite peculiar to them. They call it *rasāyana.* Rasa is gold'. Al-Biruni also refers to Nagarjuna as a famous alchemist hundred years before to him. He wrote detailed observation on India's science and technology.

Prof. P.C. Ray in his well-known book *History of Hindu Chemistry* believes that the alchemy is indigenous to India. Surprisingly the ayurvedic word *rasāyana* denotes not alchemy but geriatrics. *Rasāyana* is a way of strengthening the body's immune mechanisms to protect it from diseases. Ayurveda looks at 'old age' and 'death' as diseases. The aim of *rasāyana* is to make the human body invincible.

The *Śārangadhara samhita* has updated the pharmacopoeia of ayurveda in the 13th century AD by introducing several mercurial preparations. The *śaivism*, which got strengthened in South India at that time, has owned the philosophy of *rasatantra*, paving way for prolific literature combining *saivism, tantrism* (occult practices) and *rasavāda*. Meulenbeld in his*History of Indian Medical Literature* supposes that the *rasaśāstra* originated in South India. He quotes *Kalyanakaraka*, which belongs to 9th c. AD to prove his argument.

The import of mercury was and is on the cards because it is not available in India. During the Vijayanagara period the import of quick-silver (mercury) happened through the ports on the west coast. The import of mercury certainly stimulated the field of alchemy in South India. Use of mineral substances in ayurveda was in vogue but limited. The *rasaśāstra* made its entry into ayurveda around 8th century AD. Ayurveda*vaidyas* of the South were overwhelmed by an obsession of transmutation of mercury into gold. Surprisingly the atomic number of mercury (Hydrarginum) is 79 and that of gold (Aurum) is 80. Herbal saps can never transmutate elements. The futile efforts of making gold from base metals are still going on in India. Use of mercury in alchemy is due to its usefulness in gold mining. Mercury easily forms amalgam with gold and heating leaves gold. Therefore, Hindus thought mercury and gold are interrelated.

Notwithstanding the trials to produce gold from mercury were futile, these experiments have yielded new herbo-mineral formulations. The idea behind using herbs in transmutation was clear. The plants grow faster. If the saps of the plants are used to grow metals, that would be a great idea. Physicians of ayurveda planned to infuse good qualities of plants into metals and administer them to humans to extend the lifespan and cure difficult-to-cure diseases. Srisailam, Nagarjunakonda and Alampur are a few places in South India, where the *rasasiddhis* (expert alchemists) labored to transmutate mercury into gold. The temple floors of Alampur still bear the marks of alchemical experiments.

Sindhura aushadha is a form of mercurial medicine made using glass containers. Ayurveda physicians of Andhra region were pioneers in *sindhura aushadhas* of medicinal alchemy. *Purnacandrodaya* and *makaradhvaja* are two important medicines of ayurveda pharmacopoeia, exclusively developed in the South. *Makaradhvaja* was hailed by the ayurveda physicians as an effective aphrodisiac. *Makaradhvaja* means *manmatha* (cupid, the god of love). It contains gold, purified mercury, purified sulfur, juices of red cotton and aloe. Purified signifies raw mercury is subjected to cleansing process using cow urine and fire. Basavaraja has added camphor, nutmeg, musk, cloves and pepper to *makaradhwaja* and named it *purṇacandrodaya* (rise of the full moon). It takes two weeks to prepare this medicine.

Ayurvedic alchemy believes that *parad* (mercury) is Siva, *abhrak* (mica) is Parvati (Siva's consort), *gandhak* (sulphur) is the *raja* (menstrual blood) of Parvati. Many fanciful theories were formulated on the origin of alchemy. These beliefs originated after *Śaivism* replaced Jainism from 12th c. onwards. We have not found any evidence of import of mercury during the Indo-Roman trade. There are speculations that the mercury was introduced from China through Tibet at that time. Mercuric sulphide, which yields mercury, is known as *darada* in ayurveda. Several inscriptional and literary evidences tell *daradas* were people who lived north to the Kashmir valley. Based on description of the *Mahābhārata* and Kalhana's *Rājataranigiṇi* this kingdom is identified to be the Gilgit region in Kashmir along the river Sindhu (Indus). This route is known for trade between China and India since ancient times. Therefore, the first source of mercury could be China.

Regional variations of Ayurveda

The pan-Indianayurveda acquired regional variations with the influence of diversity in ecosystems and varied local health traditions. In the field of classical music and dance, the regional variations are pretty clear. *Odissi* dance is different from *bharata natya* and *kuchipudi* from *kathak*. This kind of diversity is also seen in architecture, sculpture, cuisine and languages. Although ayurveda appears as homogeneous kind of traditional medicine across India, it continues in several recensions (*sampradāyas*) in different parts of the subcontinent.

In the northwest India, particularly in Rajasthan and Gujarat, ayurveda physicians tend to prescribe more *rasaushadhas* (mercurial and metallic preparations). The reason for this practice is long tradition of Jainism. In Dravidadeśa, the present day Tamilnadu, where siddha medicine is popular, earthen salts are overwhelmingly used in the preparation of medicines. In the heartland of ayurveda, Uttar Pradesh and Bihar, *kāṣṭaushadhas* (herbal preparations) are preferred to mercurial or metallic preparations. In Kerala too, more herbal preparations are prescribed; however, Kerala physicians prefer fresh green herbs to dried ones. Kerala is the only region in India to have evergreen forest. In Āndhradeśa, ayurveda is a fusion of *Ātreya sampradāya* of north and *siddha sampradāyam* of south.Ayurveda in different locations developed in such a way to suit the local epidemiology. Wherever ayurveda entered it interacted with the local folklore traditions of healing.

Ayurveda entered Kerala in 5th and 6th centuries AD along with Brahmanism and Buddhism. In Kerala, the text*Aṣṭānga hridaya* was received with much acclaim. Some of the popular ayurvedic texts of Kerala, *Śahasrayogam* contain medical knowledge, not mentioned in classical texts of the *Carakasamhita* and *Suśrutasamhita*. In addition to this, the specializations such as *viṣa* *cikitsa* (treatment in poisonous conditions), *marma cikitsa* (dealing with vital points on the body) and treatment for small-pox were practiced in Kerala from an early period. Similarly, some of the ayurvedic therapeutic methods popular in Kerala such as *dhara, pizhichil, navarakizhi, sirovasthi* etc. are the results of interactions between the classical ayurveda and the local traditions. Thus, the *Keraliya*ayurvedais a regional variation of classical medicine. Kerala is a home of indispensable and irreplaceable spices that constitute the core of ayurveda pharmaceuticals. The classics of ayurveda refer to *pippali* (Piper longum) and *marica* (Piper nigrum) as very important ingredients of innumerable ayurveda preparations. Certainly these spices are significant discoveries of the tribes living in Kerala for thousands of years that eventually entered into ayurveda. The Indus civilization has contributed for the spread of spices from Kerala to other parts of the world.

Today, it is difficult to identify regional variations among ayurveda physicians because they move a great deal within India. The regional variations in ayurveda were clearly identifiable till 1950s. In Karnataka, the name of Basavaraja was more popular than Caraka till recently. In Āndhradeśa, *Bahat* and *Vaidyacintamani* were extensively followed. The names of Caraka and Suśruta were unknown to the people of South India. Now, all ayurveda colleges have uniform syllabus and pharmaceutical companies bring uniformity in prescriptions by manufacturing and marketing products useful in all corners of India. Therefore, the regional traditions of ayurveda are now coalesced.

Siddha Medicine and Ayurveda

In Tamilnadu and Pondicherry, siddha system of medicine is the most popular among the alternative systems of medicine. The siddha medicine and ayurveda share several elements of theory and practice. The siddha system of medicine, however, claims to be an independent system with thousands of years of antiquity. The word siddha means a 'divine sage' and an 'achiever' or a person free from mundane bothering. Legend tells that Agastya, the progenitor of the system hails from the north, traversed the Vindhya Mountains and settled in the south. Eighteen siddhars were said to have contributed towards the development of this medical system. Siddha literature is in Tamil language and it is practiced largely in Tamil speaking part of South India. Salts, soils, metals, animal products and herbs are used to prepare medicine in the siddha tradition. There are twenty-five varieties of water-soluble inorganic compounds called *uppu*. These are different types of alkalis and salts. There are sixty four varieties of mineral drugs that do not dissolve in water but release vapors when put on fire.

The basic principles of siddha are not dissimilar to those of ayurveda. Siddha believes in the theories of *tridoṣa* (three humors), *saptadhātu* (seven constituent factors) and the modes of diagnosis. Siddha *sampradāya* reckons only four *mahābhutas* (cosmic elements) as components of the universe. Space, *akāśa bhuta*, is not considered as an element. Siddha system thinks of ten variants of *vāta*, while ayurveda thinks only five variants of *vāta,* that regulate the physiological processes of the body. Siddha physicians do not depend on the Sanskrit language because their authentic works were written in Tamil language. This linguistic freedom has helped the scholars of Dravidadeśa to be independent and assertive.

The prevalence of salts in therapies is an indication that the siddha system has roots in the Indus civilization. The state of Punjab, with five big perennial rivers and proximity to the Himalayan region yields diverse salts on the river beds and mountain folds. Use of these salts predates the *Vedic* times, according to the siddha tradition. The siddha medicine gradually became a conglomeration of occultism (*tantra*), yoga, alchemy and herbal therapies. Siddha medicine has started taking its present form from the Cola dynasty in the 9th century AD. Marital alliances between the kings of Tanjavur in Tamilnadu and Vengi in Āndhradeśa from 10th century onwards have created favorable time for the fusion of ayurveda with southern traditions. Although ayurveda uses rock salt (*saindhavalavaṇa*), more advanced complex salts like *poner, jainer* and *amuri* are not mentioned in the ayurvedic texts.

Kenneth Zysk tried to prove the Buddhist antiquity in siddha medicine. Zysk quotes an interesting parallel between Jivaka the physician and surgeon removing worms from a head of a person in Rajagriha and a siddha physician removing a frog from head of a patient. The

Sangam literature, the earliest Tamil literature, was influenced by the Buddhist *sangha*, hence the name. Siddha has distanced itself from the northern tradition. Siddhars are venerated as gods in South India. The Palani temple near Dindigal in Tamil Nadu is associated with Bogor, where the siddhar had prepared an idol using nine *mahāviṣa* (great poisons). The consecrated water and milk collected from bathing of this idol is used as medicine. A combination of *viram* (mercuric chloride), *puram* (mercuric chloride), *rasam, jathilingam, kandagam* (sulphur), *gauri pasanam, vellai pasanam* (white arsenic), *mridharsingh*, *silasat* (bitumen) were used to make this idol.

Yunani Tibb and Ayurveda

The word yunani sounds *yavana,* which was used to refer to Greeks and later used to Persians and Arabs. The word Tibb means medicine. Therefore, yunani literally means 'foreign medicine'. The yunani system of medicine is relatively a new entrant into India. It was mainly patronized by the Islamic regimes of Delhi from 11th century AD. Its roots are in Greek, Persian and Arab systems of medicine. Royal patronage of yunani reached its pinnacle during Moghul period. The Delhi Sultanate even appointed yunani physicians in its royal court. The yunani medicine is based on the teaching of Hippocrates (5th century B.C.), Galen (2nd century AD) and Avicenna (Ibn Sina) (9th -10th centuries AD). This system got enriched by absorbing the best therapies of Egypt, Syria, Persia, India and China. After its entry into India, the Sharifi families in Delhi, Azizi family in Lucknow and Nizams of

Hyderabad have greatly patronized it. The yunani system too believes in three humoral forces, whose balance is thought to be maintaining health and imbalance leading to disease. The diagnostic methods include observing pulse (*nubz*), urine and stools along with others like external observation and temperament of the body. Yunani prefers medicines made from single herbs to compound formulations. The striking feature of yunani is its proximity to the diagnostics of ayurveda and siddha.

Islamic contacts with South India began as early as the 7th century AD, a result of trade between the southern kingdoms and Arab lands. Jumma Masjids existed in the Rashtrakuta Empire by 10th century AD and many mosques flourished on the Malabar Coast by early 14th century. Muslim settlers married local women; their children were known as *mappillas* (Moplahs) and were actively involved in horse trading and manning shipping fleets. The contacts between the Vijayanagara Empire and the Bahamani Sultanates increased the presence of Muslims in the South. Penugonda in Anantapur district is known for the presence of Muslims before the establishment of Islamic regimes in Delhi by the central Asian Islamic hoards. *Dudekula* Muslims belong to this category. Fakruddin, the Sufi saint saw the sprouting of *pilu* tree (Salvadora persica) in Penugonda and chose this place to live. The twigs of *pilu* are used as toothbrushes. As these are mostly converts, not much medical data has flown from the Middle East. After the fall of Kākatiya kingdom in Warangal, the yunani system of medicine made significant inroads into South India.

Arka, a pharmaceutical preparation made using a technique of distillation, was learned by ayurveda from the yunani system of medicine. *Arka,* a distillation technique is useful to prepare the medicine from the plants containing volatile substances. In ayurveda pharmacopoeia, the ratio of volatile herbs is very low. With the entry of this technique, utility of some plants like camphor became popular. The text *Arkaprakāśa* describes the methods to extract distillations even from non-aromatic plants. However, the number of *arkas* is very less in today's ayurveda pharmacopoeia. The Islamic conquest brought new herbs and therapies to India. Hyoscyamus (henbane) was introduced from west Asia into the Indian subcontinent. Hyoscyamus's Sanskrit name, *parasika yavani* (*ajvain*), points to its introduced nature: *parasikas* means people of Persia.

Increasing presence of yunani physicians in south, particularly in Nizam's dominion, has escalated its popularity. Dar-Us-Shifa (House of Cures) was the first hospital established in Hyderabad in 1595 AD on the southern bank of the river Musi by Sultan Mohammed Quli Qutb Shah, the founder of the city of Hyderabad. It was a two-story building with 40 rooms each of which accommodated four or more beds. Simultaneously, there was great exchange of know-how between ayurveda and yunani. Ayurveda has learned to make new preparations like *gulkand* (aphrodisiac paste made from rose petals), *jivanadhara* (made from camphor useful in respiratory disorders) etc.

State patronage is not essential for the progress of science. State cannot and does not expunge the evolving technology. The Moghul Empire has not discriminated against ayurveda; instead, there were several yunani and ayurveda hospitals across India. Ayurveda and yunani medicine received equal royal patronage. In Ain-i Akbari, Abul Fadl has listed twenty-nine prominent physicians and surgeons, both Hindus and Muslims, all of whom were on royal pay roll. Though Akbar was illiterate, he was wise enough to seek suggestions to improve the conditions for the people in his kingdom. One of his physicians, Hakeem Abul Fatah, suggested that due attention should be paid to the art of medicine, more physicians recruited and hospitals and dispensaries established. Akbar accepted this suggestion. Akbar built a large hospital at Fatehpur Sikri and another at Agra at the place where now stands the Agra fort railway station. The profession of a physician was lucrative in the Moghul period.

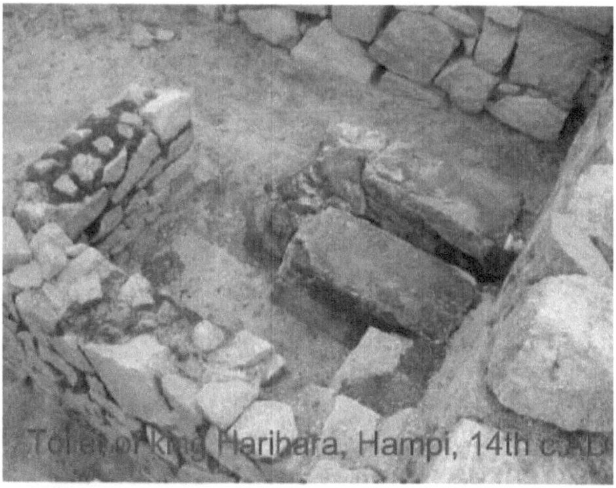
Toilet of king Harihara, Hampi, 14th c AD

Toilet of King Harihara, Hampi, South India, 14th c.AD

Chapter Four

AYURVEDA IN THE COLONIAL AGE

The worst thing that colonialism did was to cloud our view of our past.

— Barack Obama, President USA

Humans tend to move to new places. Migrations have greatly improved the quality of human life since prehistoric times. New places have provided new resources and new markets. The Indian subcontinent has witnessed a number of human incursions from all sides. However, the arrival of Europeans from 16th c. AD has altered the course of history of medicine forever.

It is not easy to mark the exact beginning of colonial period in India. Different parts of the subcontinent came under colonial administration at different times. Vasco-da-Gama, a queen's representative from Portugal, discovered a new sea-route to the spicy Konkan coast in south India. The arrival of Vasco-da-Gama on the west coast on 20th May 1498 AD hastened and expanded the trade between pre-industrialized Europe and the Vijayanagara Empire of south India. In the ensuing years, the Vijayanagara Empire, with its resplendent capital city of Hampi, has enjoyed brisk trade with Europe and Middle East. Gradually, the Portuguese have stabilized their power in Goa. The founding of the East India Company in 1600 AD in London under the Tudor rule was an epoch-making event. Slowly, but steadily, the British made efforts to expand their business in the subcontinent. The dissolution of Moghul Empire in the eighteenth century, particularly the death of Aurganzeb in 1707, is considered as beginning of the colonial rule in India. The battles of Plassey (1757) and Buxor (1764) in Bengal have given the British a chance to enjoy power in India. However, direct British rule was imposed after the Sepoy Mutiny in 1857. The French and British competed for supremacy in India but finally the sphere of influence of France shrank to Pondicherry in South India.

The seeds of European influence on Indian medicine can be traced to the period of Moghul times in the north and Vijayanagara Empire in the south. Portugal was the first pre-industrialized European nation that contacted South India. Several medical terms entered from Portuguese into South Indian languages. The linguists have identified words *aya* (dry nurse or baby sitter) and *aspatri* (hospital) in Telugu and other Dravidian languages as Portuguese in origin. Other common words like *sabbu* (soap), *tuvvalu* (towel), *chavi* (key), *almirah* (shelf) have entered Dravidian languages from Portuguese. The Portuguese introduced tobacco and red pepper (chillies). The word *batu* for duck is from Portuguese, which was used by the king Srikrishnadevaraya (1489-1529) in his poetic work *Amuktamālyada*. The diseases syphilis unintentionally introduced by the Portuguese, was referred to in the *Bhāvaprakāśa,* an important treatise of ayurveda of 16th century.

An English Factory at Machilipatnam (in Andhra Pradesh) was founded in 1611 AD; in 1613 a trading station became permanent at Surat. In

1615 the company arranged to have James I to send Thomas Roe as a royal ambassador to the court of Jahangir. The visitors have presented some gifts including a world map and a chronometer to Jahangir. These gifts were not appreciated by the Indian kings! They could not guess the world map is going to change the future of the world. James Coryut (1577 – 1617) roamed in India and died near Surat. He left an interesting account of his experiences in India. He earned the name Indian *fakir*. The British gradually established their base in Bengal and started their business in the 18th century.

The European involvement in Indian administration has helped the public health in many ways. Modern education and industrial growth have gradually increased the lifespan of the Indians. The law and order situation too has been greatly improved. The society experienced relative peace and prosperity as criminal gangs like *piṇḍaris* and *thugs* were controlled and ruthlessly punished by the British. The *thugs* were a network of devotees of goddess Kali spread throughout the subcontinent, who mercilessly killed travelers on the highways. The thugs committed murders as a religious duty and their behavior was very normal before and after their crimes. They cannot be identified by their normal conduct. Any person could become a member of this cult. It is reported that 40,000 travelers were losing their lives every year in colonial India because of thugs and more than two million innocent Indians were maimed and killed by the thugs according to the statistics collected by the British. William Henry Sleeman, a police officer in the British India has been hailed as a hero because he suppressed this barbaric cult saving the lives of the people.

India has attracted physicians, politicians, traders, merchants and treasure hunters in great numbers from European nations in the colonial age. Some of these educated and informed Europeans have left their chronicles, which reflect the life of a physician and the state of medicine in India. Their recordings are of immense help in understanding the status and progress of ayurveda. The influence of western medicine on ayurveda is visible from this period. It is surprising that ayurveda physicians could not update their knowledge in human anatomy and physiology available in the colonial times; instead, views of ayurveda on structure and function of the human body were cherished like immutable Indian *science*.

Narratives of Foreign Visitors

The transport and communications between the continents have reached a new height in the 16th century AD due to the improvements in the navigation and printing technology. Rough world maps were prepared and behavior of ocean currents was understood. Several visitors have ventured to reach India via land and sea. Many Europeans trekked on land to reach India to study the markets and improve their trade of precious stones, horses and other commercial items. Some visitors have left behind their chronicles. Their writings shed light on the status of ayurveda and the lives of ayurveda physicians. Although many of these visitors were not physicians, to objectively comment on ayurveda, their writings are useful to get a perspective on ayurveda in colonial India.

Opinions and observations of Nicolo de Conti (an Italian, who arrived in India in 1505 AD), Garcia Da Orta, (Portuguese physician, who practiced medicine for 36 years in Goa), Francois Bernier (who visited Masuilipatnam and Golkonda in 1666-67), Charles Dellon (a French Physician, who wrote two books with copious references to ayurveda), John Fryer (c. 1650–1733) offer many interesting observations on contemporary medicine.

Colloquies on simples and drugs of India was published by Garcia da Orta in Goa in 1563 AD in Latin language. Garcia da Orta was the earliest European physician in India. He came to India as a physician on Portuguese ships, and became well acquainted with native kingdoms and their medical systems. He was a physician to the Viceroy of Goa and had a garden with medicinal herbs in his compound. In his book, he refers to conversations he had with ayurveda and yunani physicians to understand their principles and modes of treatment. His book does not look into the concepts of ayurveda because he was more interested in the medicinal plants and comparing the diseases affecting people in India with the diseases affecting people in Europe. He treated Burhan Nizam Shah, ruler of Ahmednagar, for skin eruptions. Orta died in Goa in 1568 AD.

Tavernier, an Italian jewel merchant widely traveled in India wrote in 1615 AD that there were no doctors in the society except with kings. He describes the happenings at Golconda, where the sultan suffering from severe headache was in search of a surgeon to conduct bloodletting technique on him. The Sultan could take the help of a Dutch surgeon. Tavernier's recordings also reflect on the type of food the common people eat in south India.

Francois Bernier (1625 – 1688) of France was orphaned at an early age and brought up by his uncle. After studying mathematics, theology and astronomy in Paris, he studied at Montpellier medical school for just 3 months intensively. After traveling through Middle East, he reached Surat, in 1658 or 1659 A.D. He met Aurangazeb, then Moghul king of India, through a French physician and was appointed as royal physician. He witnessed several historical events of that time. He observed 'where anatomy is concerned we can say that the Hindus know nothing at all; they simply spew out impertinent nonsense. It is therefore not surprising that they are so ignorant since they never open the body of man or animal'. Bernier's observed frequent cases of filariasis and dracunculosis. He described how healers skillfully extract the worm from the leg by winding around a small stick.

Bernier died in 1688 AD. His *Voyages de François Bernier contenant la description des États du Grand Moghol* was published in 1670-1671, less than two years after his return, and was translated into English (Travels in the Moghul Empire A.D. 1657-1668). He brought Harvey's theory of blood circulation to India. When he cut open a goat to demonstrate the circulation of the blood, the people witnessing it ran away in scare. Therefore, he ridiculed the Indian sciences for their stagnation.

Charles Dellon (1650 – 1710 AD) had

visited South India and spent approximately eight years from 1668 AD to 1676 AD as a physician. He lived in Daman for some time. He observed 'From this moment onwards, I began seeing patients at the hospital and in their homes. At that time, Daman only had a few pundits, or Indian physicians, with very limited skills. The only knowledge possessed by such physicians consisted of a few remedies that they dispensed as prescribed by tradition rather than reason. Furthermore, since Europeans enjoy high esteem in the Orient, and since I was not lacking in boldness myself, my services were called upon not only by the Portuguese, but also by the Indians. As the town of Daman is not particularly large, I was soon a familiar figure everywhere'.

Charles Dellon faced the inquisition by the Portuguese and spent few years in prison in Goa. He studied hundreds of medicinal plants of India and their uses. He published a book on medicine, *Traité des maladies particulières aux pays orientaux, et dans la route, et leurs remèdes* (Treatise on the diseases specific to the Orient and travel thereto, their remedies), in Paris in 1685. Its sixty two pages deal with diseases commonly encountered during the voyage and in India itself, such as scurvy, vomiting, cholera, smallpox, snakebites, and filariasis, as well as the 'exhaustion caused by sexual excess'. In addition to extolling bleeding and purging, Dellon recommended some Indian treatments such as betel leaf, betel nut, and congee, salted ground-rice porridge in diarrhea. He has observed ayurveda physicians from close. He says 'Indian pagans, called themselves *pundits*, knew nothing of anatomy. They only inherited certain recipes'.

John Fryer of Great Britain traveled in India for nine years, between 1672 and 1681 AD. Fryer mentions of animal hospitals in India though he sharply criticizes Indian doctors are more merciful and charitable to the animals than to humans. He narrates day-to-day medical practice of Indian doctors. He notes that 'surgery – beyond amputation – is not practiced, and that leeching is used in preference to phlebotomy. They are unskilled in anatomy. Phlebotomy is not understood, they being ignorant how the veins lye; but they will worry themselves martyrs to death by leeches, clapping on a hundred at once, which they know not how to pull off, till they have filled themselves, and drop of their own accord. Chirurgery is in as bad a plight, amputation being a horrid thing: yet I confess it is strange to see, that what nature will effect on such bodies, intemperance has not debauch'd'. He continues with a criticism of pharmacists, and interestingly takes note of the preference for pulse diagnosis over urine examination.

In medieval period, the physicians did not have access to university kind of education where many physicians live in one place and interaction among them will be a major driving force for the science. In those days, every ayurveda physician was an institution by himself and exchange of information and ideas among the ayurveda physicians was not in vogue. The knowledge of ayurveda was inherited through some families. The son of a physician became a physician. Stagnation and prejudiced opinions of ayurveda scholars were main obstacles for the progress of medicine. Fryer was right in saying that there was no system of certification in ayurveda. Even today, ayurveda physician is judged by his or her oration of verses in Sanskrit and defeating opponents in verbal duels. There was no system in India to compile and standardize the inventions and discoveries in medicine at the time of Fryer's visit.

In the 18th century, Colin Mackenzie was carrying a survey in south India to collect manuscripts, inscriptions and any written records in any form. He had come across several important ayurvedic manuscripts. The Asiatic Society published this catalogue in 1828. It mentioned many ayurveda treatises written in the middle ages. Mackenzie collected several works on medicine in Tamil speaking region too. *Agastya vaidyam*, a palm leaf work with 1500 verses, *Agastya purana sutra, Bhasmamore* (a work on alchemy), *Balacikitsa, Agasta vaidya munnur, Agastya vaidya nuthiyambid, Agastya vaidya napatettu, Vaidya sutra nuru, Muppu, Terumalar vaidyam* were collected by Mackenzie.

Hortus Malabaricus (Garden of Malabar) is an exhaustive survey of medicinal plants in Kerala region. This was compiled in Latin language, and published from Amsterdam (Netherlands) during 1678-1703. It comprises 12 volumes of about 500 pages each, with 794 copper plate engravings. Over 742 different plants and their indigenous science are dealt in the book. There were several Ezhava physicians (Itty Achudan and others), who contributed to this compendium. *Hortus* certainly reflects the local flavor and knowhow of Kerala tribes. Foremost social reformer, Narayana Guru hails from Ezhava community, who fought caste discrimination and strived for social justice. He himself was a reputed ayurveda scholar. Ezhavas constitute around 23% of Kerala's population and have immense influence on medicine.

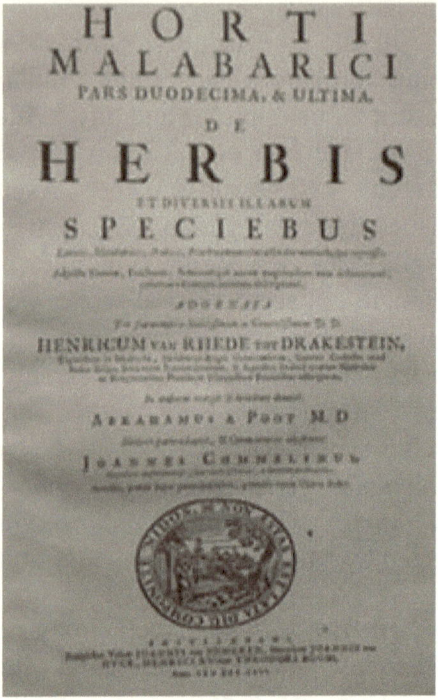

HORTI
MALABARICI
PARS DUODECIMA, & ULTIMA.
DE
HERBIS
SPECIEBUS
HENRICUM VAN RHEEDE TOT DRAKESTEIN,
M.D
JOANNES COMMELINUS

In 1881, Basel Mission in Mangalore published a book titled *Five Hundred Indian Plants-their use in medicine and arts in Canarees* with vernacular names in Kannada, Tulu, Malayalam, and Konkani. The book describes a total of 523 plants and their medicinal uses.

At the end of the 19th century, the discovery

of Bower's manuscript in northwest China (on the Silk Road) has been an important event in the study of history of ayurveda. This manuscript was acquired by Lieutenant Hamilton Bower, who was searching for a criminal in central Asia. The Bower manuscript is known as *Yaśomitrasamhita* and its scribes were Buddhists, who collected birch bark for writing media from Kashmir. Hoernle edited and published this manuscript. Now the Bower's manuscript is found in the Bodleian Library in Oxford. The scholars of 19th century had energetically collected ayurvedic manuscripts from every nook and corner of India. The scholars of ayurveda started thinking that these manuscripts hide many secrets that are being exploited by the English! The illiteracy rates were so high in India, the rumors were easily believed. The dominant castes continued their domination by their inherited snobbish psychology. The new knowledge coming from the west seems to be ineffective in modernizing the society.

Institutionalization of Ayurveda

Recovery of ayurveda has started in Bengal in the 19th century AD. Ayurveda physician is known as *kavirāja* in Bengal region. *Kavirājas* managed *Tol*, a school of ayurveda, at their residences. Students used to flock to the teacher and stay few years to learn ayurveda. Many teachers give free food and education to their students. It was the period ayurveda has not yet entered into a system of formal education from its traditional apprenticeship method. It all started in Bengal.

Natives were enrolled as subordinates into

the medical services of East India Company. A school for native doctors was founded in 1822 and from 1827 ayurveda was added to the curriculum of western medical techniques in teaching. In 1833, William Bentinck, the Governor General of British India, appointed a committee to review the medical education. Basing on the recommendations of the committee, Bengal Medical College was founded on 20th February 1835. It alienated ayurveda from modern medicine. The inauguration of the college was a celebrated event in the history of medicine in India. From then on, ayurveda was restricted to the homes of physicians. Subsequently, ayurveda returned to family traditions. The young students in Bengal, who join training in modern medical institute, were given free books, modern medical knowledge and even scholarships. Studying modern medicine was financially beneficial so the *kavirājas* too wished their sons studied modern medicine.

Some historians of medicine think that the British have snubbed ayurveda to encourage western medicine in India. However, the western medicine of that period was not yet able to compete with the traditional systems of medicine. Some progress was made in vaccination by the work of Edward Jenner. Louis Pasteur and Robert Koch are yet to discover and revolutionize medicine. At that point of time, the European physicians were recognizing the importance of hygiene in preventing epidemics. Therefore, the idea of suppression of ayurveda by the British is imaginary. The Anglicists were of the opinion that the ayurveda physicians were non-progressive and not open-minded.

Some ayurveda physicians have strived for

ayurveda sincerely. Gangadhara Ray, born in 1789 in east Bengal, studied Sanskrit and ayurveda in a *Tol* of kavirāja Ramakanta Sen. He moved to Calcutta in 1819 and practiced ayurveda. In 1835, he came to know that a modern medical college was established in Calcutta and a Brahmin student performed the first dissection on a dead human body. It is said that he left Calcutta in despair. He was an erudite scholar in Sanskrit and he worked on approximately eighty books on ayurveda. His famous commentary on *Carakasamhita* is *Jalpakalpataru*. He died in 1885. To his last breath, he was an ayurveda physician to the core. He never learned English and was not interested in western medicine.

Gangaprasad Sen was another brilliant ayurveda practitioner in Bengal. Born in 1824 at Dacca, East Bengal, Sen learned ayurveda from his father. His strength was in formulation of medicines. He was the pioneer in marketing ayurveda medicines. He wanted to compete with European medicine and he was the first person to export ayurvedic medicines to Europe and America. He started practicing ayurveda in Calcutta at the age of nineteen! He fixed his consultation fee and advertised his clinic competing with western clinics. He published an ayurvedic journal, *Ayurveda Sanjivani*, in Bengali. By the time he died in 1896, he was one of the richest persons in Calcutta. Ramakrishna Paramahamsa, the mentor of Swami Vivekananda, was one of his patients.

Bijoyratna Sen, who translated *Aṣṭāngahṛdaya* into Bengali, Chandrakishore Sen,

Gananath Sen and many other brilliant ayurveda practitioners were the products of Bengal renaissance. The hallmark of this period is self-admiration; the western medicine was viewed as a contender. Ayurveda scholars founded many pharmaceutical companies and institutes. Similar to the cultural renaissance of Bengal, this movement has spread to the rest of India. However, India did not produce a visionary like Raja Rammohan Roy in ayurveda. Therefore, the renaissance of ayurveda in Bengal remained an unfinished task.

In South India, Madras (Tamilnadu), Mysore (Karnataka), Vijayawada (Andhra Pradesh), Thiruvananthapuram (Kerala) stood ahead in founding exclusive institutes for ayurveda. These institutes were enterprises of some individual enthusiasts. Until 1880s, there was no demand for exclusive ayurveda colleges. In 1905, Sri Venkateswara Ayurveda College was founded in Madras. This college used to publish *Dhanvantari*, a journal of ayurveda in Telugu language. In 1912, the *mahants* of Tirumala (Trustees of the temple) started an ayurveda institution in Tirupati, Andhra Pradesh. In 1918, Gurukul Kangdi Ayurveda College in Uttar Pradesh and one ayurveda institution in Kasi, Uttar Pradesh were founded. In 1920, the Indian National Congress, spearheading the national movement, has affirmed its attitude towards Ayurveda. It proclaimed that separate institutions would be started for the study of ayurveda in independent India. This resolution was reaffirmed in 1938.

In Kerala, the course of ayurveda has not interacted with other parts of South India because this region is geographically isolated from the rest. Nestled between the Western Ghats and Arabian Sea, Kerala is the only place with evergreen forest. Therefore, Kerala is a paradise for ayurveda physician. Although this region was a part of Cola-Pandya-Cera kingdoms, Kerala pursued a different path. The rich plant life has helped the indigenous people like Ezhavas to become experts in herbal medicine. In Kerala, modern mode of instruction in ayurveda began with the establishment of an ayurveda school in 1889. A Department of Ayurveda was also established in the same year by the Government. Facilities for learning ayurveda existed at Thiruvananthapuram, Kottakkal, and Thrippoonithura. Titles awarded to the students differed; in Thiruvananthapuram it was *Vaidyakalanidhi*; Thrippoonithura – *Ayurveda Siromani* and *Vaidyabhushanam*; and at Kottakkal it was *Āryavaidyan*.

The elite class of the Indian society was demanding for the setting up of ayurvedic institutes. The demand was mainly coming from the traditional ayurveda physicians. Politically India was divided into provinces. The city of Calcutta was the headquarters of the British administration. Madras in the south, Bombay in the west and Delhi in the north were centers of British power. The system of diarchy in the provinces allowed local governments reflect the aspirations of the people. This system was later replaced by provincial autonomy in 1935. In the south, Koman Committee was constituted by the Madras government in 1920s to study the problems of ayurvedic education. This committee reported that it is not necessary to establish exclusive ayurveda and yunani hospitals; instead, effective therapies of traditional medicine may be introduced in modern hospitals. The Usman Committee of 1921, appointed by the Madras government, recommended greater cooperation between western and ayurveda physicians. This committee has favored separate registration for the institutionally trained and homegrown ayurveda physicians. This committee also recommended extensive use of ayurveda therapies in rural areas. In 1944, the British government has appointed a committee, Health Survey and Development Committee, also known as Bhore Committee to suggest mode of medical education for India. This committee has supported scientific medicine for the needs of India. It did not comment on ayurveda. In 1946, the government has appointed Chopra Committee to reconcile the problems of medical education, because ayurveda physicians were divided on the question of distance to keep from the western medicine.

In the south, Achanta Laxmipathi and Yellapragada Subbarao represent two different streams of thinking. Achanta Laxmipathi (1880 – 1962), trained in western medicine, has enthusiastically studied ayurveda. Achanta was a prolific writer. His encyclopedic work, *Ayurveda śikṣa*, had immensely influenced the students of ayurveda. The content of his writings is naïve, lacks scientific spirit and his overemphasis on dogma of ayurveda render him an amateur of ayurveda. He represents the purists' school of ayurveda.

Yellapragada Subba Rao born in Andhra

region in 1895 studied in Madras Medical College. He worked in Ayurveda College in Madras and taught anatomy to the students of ayurveda. He later proceeded to the United States in 1922. In America, he did a commendable job in pharmaceutical research. He invented Hetrazan (used against filariasis), developed anti-cancer drug Methotrexate, isolated folic acid etc. Subba Rao has left Ayurveda College because he thought Ayurveda College is not a place for progress! He tried to revive his interest in ayurveda while in the US and later it was clear for him that the research into ayurveda leads to dead-end.

Ayurveda at Crossroads

Ayurveda physicians in the colonial times embarked upon treating patients suffering from syphilis, which reached India through Portuguese traders in the 16th century AD. Syphilis was one of the worst epidemics of Europe that claimed millions of lives. The patients suffering from syphilis approached ayurveda physicians, who ought to find a remedy. Ayurveda physicians have first observed the signs and symptoms and tried to correlate them to *tridoṣa* theory. They tried to describe syphilis in the light of the principles of ayurveda. However, the humoral theory was not able to solve this riddle. The *Sarabharajiya* has classified this disease into eighteen varieties based on signs and symptoms according to the predominance of humors. The *Navaratnakara* describes syphilis in 12 forms. This disease spreads through sex and intimate human contact. It reached epidemic proportions in south India in 17th and 18th centuries AD. Syphilis was a big menace until the advent of antibiotics few decades ago. Although wood of *phiranga* (Papaya) was used to heal, *Siddha* medicine has succeeded marginally by using salts and minerals against syphilis. Ayurveda recommended *rasakarpura* against syphilis: however, the results were not encouraging. Every year thousands of Indians were dying because of plague, small pox, malaria and other epidemics and ayurveda was of no help. The gazetteers give us the health statistics of 19th and 20th century.

The growing Indian economy and colonial administration has driven thousands of Indians to other countries and continents as well. People moved a great deal from one place to the other within and without. Indian students visited England for studies. The British has encouraged Indian farmers to migrate to Malaysia, Java, Fiji, South Africa and South America as farm laborers. In some countries (British Guiana), Hindi has become the national language. Ayurveda too had chances to enjoy popularity in these far off places, where a large Indian Diaspora existed. For the first time in history of India, hundreds of princely states and principalities coalesced to form one nation. Having formed during the colonial period, India is a young nation, because at no time in the past, even during the rule of Asoka, the entire subcontinent was politically united. This has elevated the image of ayurveda as national medicine of India.

The British government has introduced several legislatures to control the practice of medicine. Ayurveda physicians reproached some of these laws. The Magic Remedies & Objectionable

Advertisement Act of 1954 has imposed restrictions on use of cardamom, cloves, pepper etc by the ayurveda physicians. Certain aphrodisiacs like *pancabana ras, mahakama sanjivani ras* etc were banned. The Hamdard pharmacy in Delhi has appealed to the court, which granted a provisional stay.

Andhra Ayurveda and Homoeopathic Act of 1956 directed all the ayurveda physicians and pharmacies to apply for license to make and prescribe ayurvedic medicines. Other acts that appeared hostile to ayurveda physicians were Drug Act, Spirituous Preparation Act, Medicinal Preparation and Toilet Act, Madras Prohibition Act, Intoxicant Drugs Act, Dangerous Drugs Act, Central Excise Act and Gold Control Act. Several ayurvedic products were subjected to scrutiny and taxation. Most of these laws have been enforced after the India's independence. Some progressive ayurveda physicians have accepted these acts because they help government's budget. Slowly, the ayurveda physicians started understanding the need of state control on medical administration.

During this period, increased interaction with Europeans has prompted ayurveda scholars towards further consolidation of their orthodox views. The idea of modernization suffered a setback due to ideological backlash by certain sections of Hindus against the modern medicine. Therefore, ayurveda remained unaltered throughout colonial times.

Ayurveda physicians of India, whether north or south, have not updated their knowledge and expertise of healing. The basic underpinnings of ayurveda are not tested against fresh knowledge. The concepts of *pratyakṣapramāna* (direct evidence), *anumāna pramāna* (inference), *yukti* (intelligence) and *āptavākya*(information from others) are perfectly suitable to update the knowledge of medicine, but ayurveda scholars were blind to the changes in the world. The science and scientific medicine too depend on 'direct evidence' and 'inference' to acquire knowledge. Inside structure of the human body was getting clearer and clearer year by year, but ayurveda physician did not show interest in anatomy. The data that filled the pages of English medicine was the result of *pratyakṣa, anumana* and *yukti pramāna*. When the epistemological modes are same why Indian physicians ignore the results? Why ayurveda physicians haven't refined their knowledge after the interaction with the travelers from the west? Majority of scholars in India were genuinely not interested in truth. The scientific medicine grew out of epistemology, which Indians admitted as valid way to gain true knowledge. However, they practiced in obscure comprehension. Apparently, the influence of religion and caste has come across the way of progress of medicine in India. Instead of looking at the progress of medicine using the same old concepts of epistemology, ayurveda scholars have continued with their ambiguous thinking and ignored the gulf between the theory and practice of ayurveda. Thus, the Indian scholars could not rise to the situation to work with English Orientalists, who wanted to appropriate medicine and medical education to the needs of India in vernacular languages.

Similar kind of situation existed in Europe in the middle ages due to authority of church over the intellectual heritage. However, the European scholars unshackled themselves. Paracelsus (1493 – 1541), a Swiss German physician, alchemist and botanist, burned down the Avicenna's Canon of Medicine in public and refuted the humoral theory. He replaced the humors with sulphur, mercury and salt and alchemy with chemistry. Such radical thinking and approach has changed the face of European medicine during the days of renaissance.

However, some contributions were indeed made by ayurveda to scientific medicine. The Indian technique of rhinoplasty has revolutionized the plastic surgery in the 18th century Europe. In 1739 two medical officers of East India Company reported in the Madras Gazette on the practice of rhinoplasty by a potter's community in Pune district, which later appeared in Gentlemen's Magazine. Joseph Constantine Carpue, a British surgeon, learned this technique of rhinoplasty without visiting India. He introduced this technique into Europe. Rhinoplasty is a surgical technique to reconstruct lost nose. In ancient and medieval India, it was common to sever the nose as a form of punishment for treason, cheating and corruption. Victims approached ayurveda surgeons for help. Ayurvedic surgeon had the obligation to invent a technique to give new life to those unfortunates, who lost the nose. In this creative technique, the skin of the cheeks is peeled from top, folded on to nasal area, and sutured. Subsequently, fat is deposited under the skin naturally and it thickens.

This operation will create a new nose and bestows new life to the patients. This is an original Indian invention in surgery, which gave birth to the 'plastic surgery' in 19th century Europe.

In the 19th century, anesthesia was invented. Thus, surgery combined with anesthesia started a completely new branch of plastic surgery. In the days of crude surgery with no anesthesia, providence saved the patients. Mostly patients died during the operation because of shock and blood loss; if not due to post-operative complications.

Ksharasutra, a cotton thread soaked in an alkali media, was used to knot through the probed wounds of fistula-in-ano. Ayurveda physicians consider this as an original Indian invention. However, the advent of laser and cryosurgery outmoded the *ksharasutra* technique.

Dawn of Western Medicine in India

Every culture in the world, outside Europe, started questioning 'why it could not conceive science and technology independently before Europe could accomplish?' Invention of paper and printing technology was first recorded in China, veterinary hospitals were first established in India, basic astronomical calculations were made in the Middle East, but modern science and technology are the products of European ingenuity.

Cohesive teamwork was the foundation on which the modern science and technology grew. The people living in Europe are geographically conditioned to give birth to science and technology. The climate in Europe during the most part of the year is favorable to do hard work. Inventions and discoveries since the Italian renaissance have resulted in new approach in all sectors of life. Adventurous maritime voyages, invention of printing and curiosity have helped the European mind to look at the nature with a fresh look. That was the period of reason and discovery. Moreover, Europe suffered terrible epidemics and wars in its history. The bubonic plague (Black Death) ravaged Europe in the 14th century and one third of its population perished. Europeans too depended on herbs for their health needs. In winter, most of the trees loose foliage and the people could not prepare herbal medicines. Samuel Hahnemann, the founder of Homoeopathic medicine, invented a new technique to preserve the herbal products for winters. The industrialization has given marvelous tools to heal the diseases. The scientific temper has given the courage to question old beliefs in medicine. By the 16th century, European physicians started considering human body equivalent to a machine that is governed by physical laws. In the beginning, modern medicine adopted the empirical treatments of the past. It looked to other cultures and continents for treatments of incurable diseases. The Quinine, derived from the bark of South American tree, is effective against malaria. Adrenaline, a neurotransmitter and cardiac stimulant, was derived from a plant ephedra used in traditional medicine of Europe.

William Harvey proved the circulation of blood in the human body in 1628. He showed the difference between the arteries and veins and demonstrated the heart as a pumping machine.

Edward Jenner's experiments in vaccination yielded fruits in 1796. The cowpox germs were injected into humans to protect them from small pox. Scientists realized the importance of hygiene. Louis Pasteur (1822 - 1895) proved that the living organisms were responsible for fermentation. The microscope helped to see the bacteria. Pasteur proved that bacteria cause anthrax and rabies. Robert Koch identified the bacteria responsible for tuberculosis and cholera. These were the epoch-making events in the history of medicine in the 19th century. Isolating insulin by Banting and Best, development of anesthesia, sulpha drugs, penicillin and other important discoveries have revolutionized the scientific medicine. Ayurveda physicians in India have not participated in this process of evolution of scientific medicine in the 19th and 20th centuries.

The invention of cowpox inoculation by Edward Jenner (1749 – 1823) to prevent the dreadful small pox in England is one of the greatest triumphs of the modern medicine. The Englishmen brought this vaccination to India 1802. However, many Indians resisted this practice. They suspected that the English were branding the Indians to send them to other continents as labor or to conscript into army. Some ayurveda physicians thought this technique of inoculating humans with cowpox lymph is not new to ayurveda. Some hymns were composed in Sanskrit language and propagated to make believe that Jenner's discovery is already known to ayurveda. However, the British could successfully inoculate vulnerable populations of India and reduced mortality rate. Later research revealed that the British themselves encouraged and composed the hymns in Sanskrit to popularize the vaccination in India. The Sanskrit hymn describing the process of inoculating cowpox lymph into humans was crafted in the first part of the nineteenth century. After a century, in the beginning of 20th century, there was controversy on this issue. Articles were published in Madras Courier and other important journals claiming that vaccination was first discovered in India. This news was seriously undermining the credit given to Jenner. However, researchers proved that the Sanskrit phrases referring to cowpox inoculation were indeed composed after Jenner's discovery. Cowpox virus does not exist in India; therefore, discovery of vaccination against small pox in India prior to Jenner is far from truth.

Ayurveda physicians pray to the Lord Dhanvantari. The treatises of ayurveda are sacrosanct. While the modern science had come off the religion, ayurveda's bond to religion is still strong. The yunani medicine is mostly admired and professed by the Islamic populations. Surprisingly, the Western medicine or Modern medicine does not carry the religious baggage of Christianity; however, it is often referred to as 'English medicine'. The Modern medicine or Western medicine is now known as scientific medicine. It reached the Indian subcontinent in the colonial times along with other burgeoning sciences and social reforms.

The modern medicine was penetrating into all corners during the colonial period as new outposts of Britain came up both in the east and the west of India. In the beginning, the English physicians were confined to ships and factories. John Woodall (1556-1643 AD) was appointed Surgeon General to the English East India Company. He authored a guide useful to surgeons, *Surgeon's Mate*. In the *Surgeon's Mate*, much emphasis is found on treating the scurvy with the fresh fruits and lime. Jacobus Bontius (1592-1631 AD) was a Dutch physician, who wrote the first book on tropical diseases.

British government has introduced certain measures to stop the communicable diseases and epidemics from taking the toll. The promulgation of the Quarantine Act of 1825 for isolation of the patients suffering from communicable diseases, the Vaccination Act enforced from 1880 and the Birth and Death Registration Act of 1896, the Epidemic Diseases Act in 1897 were important landmarks in the history of western medicine in India. The British government organized the medical services to provide facilities for medical relief and improvements in public health. These services consisted of the Indian Medical Service, the Central and Provincial Medical Services, and the Subordinate Medical Service. The members of the Indian Medical Service were recruited by a competitive examination in London until 1914, while the staff for the Central, Provincial and Subordinate Medical Services was recruited from India.

There was a bitter dispute between the British Orientalists and Anglicists on the content of education given to Indians. British Orintalists supported old Indian culture and Anglicists wished to supplant it. After prolonged disputes over the issue, the Anglicists were victorious. A new medical college was founded in 1835. To celebrate their triumph Lord Macaulay ordered a canon salute of fifty rounds to be fired from Fort Williams in Calcutta when an Indian student performed the first dissection on a cadaver in the new college.

The first medical college in Calcutta was an institute for native doctors to train in medical techniques to help the army. This institute, after running for ten years, was transformed into a modern medical college. Thus, the Calcutta Medical College became the first medical college in India. In South India Madras Medical College was the first of its kind and second in the subcontinent. The Government General Hospital in Madras was started on 16th November 1664 as a small hospital to treat the sick soldiers of the East India Company. It was located at Fort St. George. In 1772, the hospital was moved to the present location. The personnel trained in this hospital were posted to various dispensaries in the Madras Presidency. The training was given in diagnosis, treatment and preparation of medicines. In 1827, Dr. D.Mortimar was appointed as the superintendent of the hospital. A private medical hall run by Dr. Mortimar was designated as a medical school, which was opened by Sir Fredrick Adams, the then Governor of Madras on 2nd February 1835. This medical school was attached to the general hospital.

In 1842, the hospital started taking Indians as faculty. In the next two decades, the teaching staff had increased, the duration of the course extended and the curriculum was made comprehensive. The government granted 'college status' to this school on 1st October 1850 and it became Madras Medical College. In subsequent years Madras Medical College has admitted women students too and some of the women doctors became famous by rendering gynecological services.

The Nizam rulers stood ahead of others in spreading modernity in the south. Nawab Nasir-Uddaula Bahadur Nizam IV, the then king of the Hyderabad state, impressed by Dr. William McAllen, founded Hyderabad Medical College in Hyderabad in 1846. William Mc Allen's lectures on modern medicine were being translated into Urdu in the classrooms of the new medical college, while he was lecturing. Medical education in vernacular languages was unthinkable at that time. However, the English was adopted as medium of instruction in 1884. Again, in 1926-27 the medium of instruction was changed to Urdu, which was again reverted to English in 1948-49. Thus, the city of Hyderabad served as gateway for the modern thoughts in medicine.

The Portuguese founded the Goa Medical College in 1842 in the name of *Escola Medico-Cirurgica de Goa*. Western medicine was taught in Portuguese language for more than one hundred years. The medium of education was changed to English in 1962, when the territory of Goa came under Indian administration. Krishnarajendra Wodeyar started a Medical College in 1924 in Mysore, which was the capital of erstwhile Mysore state.

The pharmacopeias and materia medica of

those days contained mostly galenicals (of Galen) and inorganic chemical preparations. The raw materials like cinchona bark, nux vomica seeds, poppy pods etc, were shipped from India to England and returned as extracts or tinctures for the physicians' use. At the turn of the century, in 1901, Acharya P.C. Ray started the first Indian-owned drug factory, the Bengal Chemical and Pharmaceutical Works near Calcutta.

The contributions of Edward Jenner (1749 – 1823) and Louis Pasteur (1822 – 1895) have offered new insights into pathology. Soon many British medical scientists researched on tropical diseases in India, which were causing much causality in the army. They established Haffkine Institute at Bombay in 1904, King Institute of Preventive Medicine in 1904 in Madras, Central Research Institute at Kasauli in 1905 and Pasteur Institute at Conoor in 1907. During the Second World War, many allopathic drugs were introduced into India. The Drug Act of 1940 was enacted. The sulphonamides, penicillins, streptomycin, tetracyclines, cortico-steroids were introduced subsequently. This has greatly helped the Indian masses to get rid of pain and suffering. In those days, many Indian men suffering from prostate gland enlargement and using catheters were experiencing infection and painful death. Pain killers and penicillin have greatly reduced the mortality rate in India.

Medical administration was divided between the centre and provinces. At the centre, the head of the medical service was director general of the Indian Medical Service, who was also medical adviser to the central government. In the provinces, medical administration was under a minister responsible to provincial legislature. The technical head of the service was designated the Surgeon-General in three provinces of Bombay, Madras and Bengal. In districts, a civil surgeon was the administrator as well as chief medical officer. In addition to this, railways and defense services had their own medical units.

The Director-General of the Indian Medical Service was in charge of medical education and higher medical services in big cities and towns. It consisted of a civil branch, a research branch, foreign and political branch and a military branch. The officers on the civil side, amounting to a third of the total cadre, were considered as war reserves. The Government of India Act, passed in 1935, reserved certain selected posts in civil branch of the Indian Medical Service for Europeans.

It was in the year 1919, the departments concerned with public health, sanitation and vital statistics were transferred to provinces. This was the first stage of decentralization of Health Administration. In 1935, the Government of India Act divided health activities under three heads; federal, provincial and concurrent, respectively, under the control of the central, provincial and central-cum-provincial governments. Health Survey and Development Committee was appointed during the Second World War. This committee, headed by Sir Joseph Bhore, submitted its report in 1946. He made a detailed survey of nation's medical and health services and made recommendations with far-reaching nature.

In 1910s, the statistics of patients visiting modern dispensaries and ayurveda and yunani dispensaries showed that ayurveda was still heading the list. South India, particularly Hyderabad, has contributed path-breaking discovery in medicine; identifying malaria parasite in a mosquito by Ronald Ross, an English physician. Use of chloroform as anesthetic was also a pioneering invention in the Osmania Medical College in Hyderabad. Ayurveda was gradually pushed to second place by the English medicine in the later part of the 20th century AD. This happened not because of discrimination by the British government but due to non-participation of ayurveda physicians in the progress of medicine.

Unfinished Blending

In spite of its coexistence with yunani, homoeopathy and western medicine, ayurveda maintained its aloofness. Ayurveda was kept deliberately away from change during the colonial period on the pretext that it was a *science* in itself. The 'scientists' of ayurveda created the prevailing public opinion on medicine. When India faced growing modern medicine, no progressive thinker of ayurveda has taken the cause of ayurveda to blend it with the changing world. We have a role model to learn from. The transformation of tradition into modernity was smooth in Japanese culture and medicine.

In Japan, modernization of medicine happened simultaneously with hastened social reforms in second half of the 19th century. Whereas Japan has not lost political independence by closing its borders to European powers, India has welcomed the foreign powers. The Meiji restoration has radically transformed the Japanese society after 1860s. No such social or political transformation has happened in India; therefore, the status of ayurveda has become a cause of concern in health sector.

In ancient Japan, treatment and prevention were based largely on religious practices, such as prayers, incantations, and exorcism; at a later date drugs and bloodletting were also employed. Chinese influence on Japanese medicine is as old as their political relations. In 7th century AD, Japanese students were sent to China to study medicine. In 982 AD, Tamba Yasuyori completed the 30-volume *Ishinho*, the oldest Japanese medical work. The concept of Yin and Yang of China is evident in this work. In 1570 AD, Menase Dosan published a fifteen-volume medical work. In the *Keitekishu* (a manual of the practice of medicine), diseases were classified and described in 51 groups. Another distinguished physician and teacher of the period, Nagata Tokuhun, whose important books were the *I-no-ben* (1585) and the *Baika mujinzo* (1611), held that the chief aim of the art of medicine was to support the natural force in the human body.

Western ideas on medicine were introduced into Japan in 16th century by Jesuit missionaries and in 17th century by Dutch physicians. Translations of European books on anatomy and internal medicine were made available in 18th century, and in 1836, an influential Japanese work on physiology appeared. In 1857, a group of Dutch-trained Japanese physicians founded a medical school in Edo

(Tokyo). Although the scientific medicine was not indigenous to Japan, important medical breakthroughs were made by the Japanese, among them the discovery of the plague bacillus in 1894, the discovery of a dysentery bacillus in 1897, the isolation of adrenaline (epinephrine) in crystalline form in 1901, and the first experimental production of a tar-induced cancer in 1918. This kind of adaptation to modernity has not happened in India during the colonial times, although a Noble prize in medicine was bagged by an English man for his work on malaria in South India.

The Japanese humorously admit that Japan failed in music and medicine! The transition from traditional medicine to modern medicine was swift and smooth in Japan. Modern ideas were integrated into the society with ease. The reaction of traditionalists to modern medicine in India was animosity and awe. Because of colonial psychology in caste-ridden society, modern medicine was not able to rudder the course of ayurveda in an appropriate and pragmatic path.

The idea of modernizing ayurveda had not picked up during the last two centuries. Many ayurveda physicians have wrong concepts on modernization. Although several articles appeared in many progressive vernacular journals like *Bharati*, a Telugu literary magazine in 1930s and 1940s, introducing new concepts of chemistry and biology to modernize ayurveda, they have not stimulated any change in the years to come. The situation was similar in all parts of the country. Blending of old with new was not initiated.

Entry of new herbs, nuts, seeds, grains, fruits and vegetables has increased diversity in food. Humans are the swiftest animals on this planet. In spite of long distances and hostile territories, human groups have been transplanting several species of animals and herbs from one habitat to the other. During the colonial times, this movement was more vigorous. Although no new significant discoveries (domestication of plant and animal species) were made during the last five centuries, hundreds of edibles have found new destinations on the map of the world. The colonial period has also helped many vegetables, fruits and grains native to small territories in India to spread to other regions. Wheat was not popular among the South Indians. During the colonial period, it gained acceptance in the South. The leavened bread is another example, which was unknown in India, has become a staple food in several families for breakfast. The bread was first introduced into the Indian hospitals as diet for the patients.

Tomato, groundnut, tobacco, carrot, red pepper, apple and many more were introduced into India. It is unbelievable that clove (Eugenia caryophyllata) and nutmeg (Mrystica fragrans) are both introduced into India in the second half of nineteenth century from Sumatra. However, the clove was mentioned in the *karpuradivarga* of the *Bhāvaprakāśa*. It is not surprising that some herbs mentioned in ayurveda treatises are not available in India. Many popular herbs in ayurveda *yaṣṭimadhu* (Sweet flag), *hing* (Asafoetida)) are not grown in India. Afghanistan is known for *hingu* and *yaṣṭimadhu* is native to central Asia. *Kumāri* (Aloe vera), opium (Papavar somniferum), *yavāni* or *ajvain*, etc. entered India not long ago and were not known to Caraka or Suśruta.

It is generally believed that Europeans introduced coffee into India. In fact, the Arabs introduced coffee into India. In 1616 AD, Edward Terry described *Cohha* and in 1700 AD. Alexander Hamilton talks of sharing 'a dish of coffee' with a Nawab. A Muslim, Baba Budan travelled to Mecca on a pilgrimage in 1720 AD and brought back few coffee seeds and started growing them near Chikmagalur, his home, in the state of Karnataka. These hills are named after him. Later, the British have cleared some tracts in the Western Ghats and cultivated coffee. Now this area grows more than 50% of coffee India produces every year. However, the habit of coffee in India has picked up due to British. The tea too was popularized because of the British. Apple plantations in Kashmir and Himachal, tea plantations in Assam, Karnataka and Kerala are living legacy of British vision.

Today's Indian lifestyle is totally influenced by the science and technology. The people demand all comforts that science can provide but they are little inclined to change the mindset. The blending of western and eastern lifestyles is happening in India but the proper blending of ayurveda and scientific medicine is still a long way. Ayurveda and the scientific medicines were not blended during the colonial period and this gulf has become a burden on the government and people now. The projection of ayurveda as a sacred cow is not going to help either economy or heritage of India.

Until the colonial age, ancient texts of ayurveda were available to very few scholars due to scarcity of writing material. The printing of books happened during the colonial period. In spite of some initial resistance, the publication of treatises and journals of ayurveda on paper hastened the process of democratization in medical education. India's independence in 1947 allured many Indians to real cultural, political, social and economic independence based on indigenous science and technology and inherited tradition, but their dreams are grounded as time passes by.

Chapter Five
AYURVEDA TODAY

Formerly, when religion was strong and science weak, men mistook magic for medicine; now, when science is strong and religion weak, men mistake medicine for magic.

---Thomas Szasz

India is a land of medical pluralism. The government of India has established exclusive medical colleges and hospitals for ayurveda, yunani, yoga, naturopathy, siddha and homoeopathy systems of medicine besides huge establishment for scientific medicine. Amid such wide range of alternatives, there is no mechanism to guide the patients to an appropriate system of medicine at appropriate time.

Ayurveda is the second biggest medical establishment after the western medicine. India governs 240 ayurveda colleges and turns out approximately 10,000 ayurveda physicians every year. The share of fiscal budget of the government of India for ayurveda is gradually increasing. The coverage of print and electronic media about ayurveda is steadily expanding. Indian companies export ayurveda medicine to other continents in large volumes. Ayurveda commerce is brisk. An ayurvedic multinational firm is recently figured in the list of black money hoarders in foreign banks!

Hundreds of new blogs and web pages appear every day to propagate ayurveda. More than 3500 pharmaceutical industries, small and big, produce tones of ayurveda medicines every year in India. *Pancakarma* and ayurveda massage centers are attracting even the healthy people to India. More people now than earlier know the word 'ayurveda'. The liberalization and globalization have been strengthening the economy of India during the last two decades. Consequently, the proportion of degenerative diseases (diabetes, stroke, cancer etc.) is rising along with the incidence of contagious (gastro-enteritis, pox etc.) diseases in India. Ayurveda is weak in containing the contagious diseases. Many patients suffering from chronic diseases like diabetes, cancer and respiratory diseases turn to ayurveda. Therefore, the modern times appear favorable to physicians of ayurveda.

The impact of globalization has created worldwide clientele base to ayurveda physicians. Several westerners admiring Indian culture are looking at 'meditation movements', ISKCON (Harekrishna movement), Yoga, *Jagadgurus* ('gurus of the world' or religious teachers from India in saffron-colored robes) and India's traditional medicine, ayurveda. Surprisingly, these cultural 'ambassadors' of India strive to visit affluent nations of the east and west instead of the indigent nations in Africa or Central America! Ayurveda physicians are optimistic and hopeful. They are unaware of real history of ayurveda and are inventing new one. They try to impress us that India's traditional medicine is pristine, pure, and scientific. This view is sponsored by some right-wing fanatics and naïve idealists, some 'upper caste elite' and some psychologically unemployed.

Commenting on the age of ayurveda,

Dominik Wujastyk says '…extravagant claims that ayurveda dates from thousands of years BC can be firmly discounted. Such claims are frequent, and arise from nationalism, religious fundamentalism, a partisan attachment to romantic ideas of India's spiritual heritage, and other such causes. They are not supported by scholarly historical research. Likewise, several English translations, intending to glorify India's past achievements, only make it seem ridiculous by falling into the trap of presenting ancient and medieval Indian medicine as though it foreshadowed all modern discoveries. Ayurveda's real history is impressive enough and does not benefit from proleptic scientism'.

Ayurveda physicians in India are divided on number of issues. Therefore, it is worthwhile to review what is happening in the field of ayurveda. Not just institutionally qualified ayurveda physicians, many botanists, religious gurus, teachers of meditation and even journalists are giving consultation to patients. Several television channels broadcast programs on ayurveda and yoga, which promise you total recovery from HIV, cancer and all incurable diseases! There are hundreds of practitioners across the country, not trained in the institutes, treat patients suffering from specific diseases like cancer, paralysis etc. Every village in India has a local therapist, who treats minor health problems from indigestion to whitlow. In metropolitan cities, many yoga and meditation teachers use the name of ayurveda to attract clientele. All this happens because the word ayurveda is not protected by copyright. Anybody can use the word ayurveda for advertising soaps, shampoos and beverages.

Ayurveda sounds magical to many. A divine feeling is associated with it. Several multinational companies entered ayurveda to expand their base of clientele. Nobody has patience and energy to impartially analyze the history, contribution, philosophical base of ayurveda to examine its claim to stand as an independent medical system.

Ayurvedic Education in India

After 1947, ayurveda physicians as well as citizens of India anticipated greater patronage for ayurveda in independent India. The Chopra committee, commissioned by the British, has submitted its report on 28th July 1948. It favored integrated approach. In the integrated approach, physicians are trained in ayurveda and western medicine. In the hospitals and rural dispensaries, the physicians of ayurveda and allopathy work together, to deliver health services on equal social status. Many physicians in India have disagreed with these recommendations. Some ayurveda physicians wanted to be *suddha ayurveda vaidyas* (pure ayurveda physicians). Majority of physicians trained in the western medicine too did not like to work with ayurveda physicians. Before implementing these recommendations, the government has appointed three more committees, Dave committee of 1956, Udupa committee of 1958 and Vyas committee of 1962-63. Udupa committee has recommended post-graduation courses in ayurveda. The Vyas committee of 1962-63 has recommended teaching and practice of *sudda* (pure) ayurveda. The parallel models of approach, i.e.

physicians trained in any system of medicine are advised to stick to their systems. The government of India ratified this policy. In 1971, the Central Council of Indian Medicine (CCIM) was established by an act of parliament. The CCIM is the apex body governing the ayurvedic medical education in India and it reports to the department of AYUSH (Ayurveda, Yoga, Yunani, Siddha and Homeopathy). The department of AYUSH is a wing of the ministry of Health of the central government. Although homoeopathy is not part of Indian systems of medicine, there are more homeopathy physicians in India than anywhere else in the world. Yunani physicians are popular among Muslim settlements. Siddha physicians are largely concentrated in the southern Indian state of Tamilnadu. In all respects, ayurveda is the biggest branch of CAM systems in India.

The main objectives of the Central Council are:

- to prescribe minimum standards of education in Indian systems of medicine viz. ayurved, siddha, yunani tibb.
- to advise Central Government in matters relating to recognition (inclusion/withdrawal) of medical qualification in/from second schedule to Indian Medicine Council Act, 1970.
- to maintain a Central Register on Indian Medicine and revise the register from time to time.
- to prescribe standards of professional conduct, etiquette and code of ethics to be

observed by the practitioners.

Today, India runs around 240 ayurveda medical colleges and one-fourth of them impart ayurveda courses at post-graduate level. Ayurveda colleges are more concentrated in western India, in the states of Karnataka and Maharashtra. Half of the Ayurveda colleges in India are located in these two regions. Ayurveda physicians both institutionally trained and those with ayurveda as family tradition elect most of the members of the CCIM. The universities and the federal government nominate some members of the CCIM.

Ayurveda colleges in India offer five and half year course in ayurveda, known as Bachelor of Ayurvedic Medicine and Surgery (B.A.M.S.). The medium of instruction in several north Indian ayurveda colleges is Hindi. Majority of colleges in south India teach ayurveda in English. Other vernacular languages like Marathi, Gujarati, Assamese, Bengali, and Oriya are also being used to teach ayurveda. Andhra Pradesh, Karnataka and Tamilnadu have founded medical universities to administer all medical courses including western medicine and courses in AYUSH. Indian Council for Cultural Relations (ICCR) of the government of India sponsors students from other countries to ayurveda colleges, which impart ayurveda education through English.

There is a scarcity of translations of treatises and reference books with standardized technical glossary of ayurvedic terms. Most of the ayurvedic terms of Sanskrit are used without change in the vernacular languages. Therefore the students understand the Sanskrit terms of ayurveda without difficulty. However, their ability to express the concepts of ayurveda in English is poor. Foreign students coming to India to study ayurveda find it difficult to understand ayurveda taught in English.

The Sanskrit remains as library language in ayurvedic education. Very few ayurveda physicians are proficient in Sanskrit language. The traditional ayurveda physicians think that it is one of the prime reasons for the reported poor quality of ayurvedic education in India. Scores of reference books of ayurveda are being published in English. There is a flood of popular ayurveda books in vernacular languages of India. But it's very difficult to find scholarly stuff among them. Most of the books published every year are mere repetitions of old books or compilations with attractive titles sans creativity. Several textbooks and reference books of ayurveda do not contain indices.

The syllabus for the Bachelor of Ayurvedic Medicine and Surgery (B.A.M.S.) course is uniform throughout India. This syllabus is prepared mimicking the subject division of the western medicine. The division of the topics and approach in teaching of ayurveda in ancient India was different from the method of teaching ayurveda today. The curriculum of ayurveda is designed in the lines of modern medical education. The division of topics into three broad categories, pre-clinical, para-clinical and clinical, is obvious to teach medicine. The pre-clinical topics include biochemistry, anatomy and physiology. The para-clinicals include pharmacology, social medicine, forensic medicine etc. The clinical subjects include surgery, medicine, gynecology, obstetrics etc. The division of ayurveda topics in B.A.M.S. course is similar to that of the modern medicine, although we do not find such division in teaching tradition of ayurveda in ancient India.

In the first year course of BAMS, *śarira racana* (anatomy), *śarira kriya* (physiology), *padārthavijñana* (physics & epistemology) including*Ayurveda itihasa* (history of Ayurveda), and Sanskrit language are taught. All these subjects are pre-clinical in nature. In the second and third years, *dravyaguṇa* and *rasaśāstra* (pharmacognacy and pharmacy), *svasthavritta* (social and preventive medicine), *agadatantra* (toxicology and medical jurisprudence), and *nidāna* (pathology) are taught. These are para-clinical subjects. In the final part of 18 month course, the students are taughtclinical subjects; *kāyacikitsa* (internal medicine), *śalya* (general surgery) *śalākya* (ENT, ophthalmology and Dental science) and *prasutistriroga* along with *bālaroga* (gynecology, obstetrics and pediatrics).

Authentic writings of ayurveda are in Sanskrit language, so the students of ayurveda are exposed to the classical treatises in BAMS course. In the first year, *Aṣṭāngahṛdaya sutrasthana* is introduced. In the second and third years the *Carakasamhita* isintroduced to the students. The student is expected to have a general view on the content and arrangement of chapters in these two treatises.

Kāyacikitsa (reparation of the body) is internal medicine. It employs medicines made from herbs, minerals and animal products along with dietary prescriptions. *Kāyacikitsa* also includes *daivavyapāśraya* (healing through prayers) and *satvāvajaya* (immuno-modulation and will power). The specialists of *śalya* deal with diseases, which are amenable to knife, fire, alkali or leeches. Surgeons of ayurveda employ methods of bloodletting using leeches and cauterization, grafting, wound healing etc. The *śalākya* specialists try to heal surgical diseases of the head, i.e. diseases of eye, ear, nose and mouth including teeth. *Prasuti stri bālaroga* specialists deal with diseases of women and children. They are obstetricians, gynecologists and pediatricians. This branch deals with both surgery and medicine. The importance of *graha* (celestial sphere or disease causing demons) is given due emphasis in *bālaroga*.

Dravyaguṇa is the study of medicinal plants and animal products like milk, ghee, urine etc. and their use in pharmacy. *Rasaśāstra* and *Bhaiṣajyakalpana* deal with the mercurial and metallic formulations. *Bhaiṣajyakalpana* means pharmacy or formulation of medicines. While the students of modern medicine do not study the processes of manufacturing medicines, the students of ayurveda study not only pharmacology in ayurveda but also ayurvedic pharmacy. *Svasthavritha* literally means 'regimen of a healthy person'. It describes the daily and seasonal regimen to help stay fit. The moral conduct too is justifiably emphasized to keep up health. *Agadatantra* is science of poisons. It classifies the plant and animal toxins and interprets their actions on the human body.

This unconventional division of topics in ayurveda appeared in the 20th century, because India wanted to adopt a parallel model for ayurveda and western medicine. The classical division of ayurveda is known as *Aṣṭānga* (eight branched) ayurveda; *kāyacikitsa, śalyacikitsa, śalākya cikitsa, stri prasuti roga, agadatantra, graha cikitsa, rasāyana and Vājikaraṇa.* Ayurveda teachers have collated various portions of ayurveda treatises and prepared tailor made textbooks for students. There is lot of ambiguity and repetition in this division of topics. To add to the confusion, the student is also exposed to some modern subjects like anatomy and physiology.

Ayurveda treatises start with examination of the patient, description of diseases, diet and treatment. The new approach of ayurvedic education, adopted by the present-day ayurveda colleges, deceptively appears refined and modern. All subjects have a fair proportion of modern topics. For instance in *śarira rachana* and *śarira kriya*, the basic knowledge of modern anatomy and physiology is given to the student. But biochemistry is not included. In *agadatantra*, the knowledge of new chemical poisons and postmortem examination is added in the curriculum. However, ayurveda surgeons are not allowed to conduct post-mortems on cadavers. The modern topics were added not to 'modernize' ayurveda, but to help the student of ayurveda to have a better understanding of the disease process and refer the patients to appropriate specialist at appropriate time. However, the revised curriculum is tempting the scholars to do syncretic interpretations of ayurvedaconcepts.

The doctors trained in new ayurveda colleges are not aware of the fact that this subject division isn't historical. The recent classification of the ayurvedic topics into clinical, para-clinical and clinical mimics the scientific medicine. New genre of ayurveda physicians specialized in preventive medicine, forensic medicine, human physiology etc. have now appeared but they are half-baked and are not trained in basic sciences and research methodologies.

Earlier (up to the first half of the 20th century), ayurveda colleges used to impart education basing on just any one of the treatises, *viz.* the *Carakasamhita*, the *Basavarājīyam*, the *Yōgaratnākaram,* with emphasis on Sanskrit language. Their knowledge of modern anatomy, physiology and pathology used to be very poor or non-existent. Nevertheless, they did not feel deficiency because ayurveda does not employ such knowledge in treatment. Apparently, the fresh knowledge of modern medicine is not giving a new perspective to ayurveda physicians.

Evidently, majority of the students, who join the BAMS courses across the country, pursue ayurveda medicine because they could not procure admission in the modern medical colleges. After the graduation in ayurveda, they feel dejected for many reasons. First, they do not have confidence in their knowledge to treat patients, because the teachers were not inspiring or motivating. Secondly, sophistication is lacking in the practice of ayurveda.

Another reason for the lack of glamour in the practice of ayurveda is lower market value of ayurvedic medical graduate. Ayurvedic graduates are ill equipped and suffering from inadequate practical knowledge and clinical skills. The social status of the ayurveda physician too is low. Some scholars think 'Unless the theory-oriented and textbook-oriented teaching is not transformed into clinically oriented practical training, the problem is probably not going to be solved'. However, nobody knows how to do it, including the CCIM.

National Academy of Ayurveda

National Academy of Ayurveda (Rashtriya Ayurveda Vidyapeeth - RAV) was established in 1988 with a major objective of promoting knowledge of ayurveda. It started regular functioning since 1991. The organization has initiated a course of MRAV (Member of RAV) in an effort to revive the traditional method of *gurukula* (hermitage) system of informal education to the graduates of ayurveda. Many believe that some important subjective knowledge of ayurveda still lies outside the ayurvedic educational institutions because, since ancient days the practicing physicians kept for them many formulations, therapies etc. and bequeathed them to their children. To bring such unshared knowledge into open access, the government of India is trying many strategies. One of such projects is RAV's plan to send students to some traditional gurus.

RAV publishes books, organizes seminars, reorientation training programs for ayurveda teachers, interactive sessions for teachers and students (because the students of ayurveda scarcely ask doubts in the classroom!) on various topics related to ayurveda. The activity of RAV is academic in nature, while CCIM is administrative. After examining the published material related to the interactive seminars and symposia, it is evident that the quality of knowledge of ayurveda scholars and the students is so poor that there is no hope of either the student or the teacher is benefited, intellectually, from the RAV.

Ayurvedic Pharmacopeia Committee

One of the most useful and accomplished organizations working for ayurveda is the Pharmacopeia Committee, established in 1962. This committee was established to compile and document various pharmaceutical formulations, including single herb medicines in various parts of the country, to assess the range of ayurvedic medicine and to bring homogeneity and uniformity in practice.

There were 22 scholars in the committee given the task of compiling official Formulary in 2 parts. In the first part single herbs, their identity is described and therapeutic values are standardized. The second part deals with compound preparations of ayurveda. Such formulary would bring uniformity in identifying herbs, preparing formulations and their therapeutic use in different pathological conditions. The formulary will set the standards for identity, purity and quality. After almost half a century of its functioning, the committee is successful in publishing highly useful material in several volumes. This data is also made accessible free on the internet. The output of this committee is highly commendable.

The 5 volumes of The Ayurvedic Pharmacopeia of India describe 418 medicinal herbs used in ayurveda. The description is about plants' identity, its names in India's vernacular languages including English, Sanskrit and botanical name, therapeutic uses and chemical constituents in brief. This kind of work is desirable in ayurveda. The APC also published another set of volumes about the formulary of ayurvedic medicines, which are not available on the net. These books are highly useful to the practicing ayurveda physicians. The work of APC is in the right direction.

Skills and Hierarchies

It is apparent that a student who completes ten years of general education will take up study of special subjects. In India, after ten years of common and compulsory (!) education, at the age of 15, students enter a two year pre-university course. They choose either biological sciences or social sciences. The successful students of biological sciences at 'plus two level' are eligible to join the 5 and half year BAMS course. In many regions a common entrance test decides whether the student joins western medicine, ayurveda or any other course. The graduate-level ayurveda course has 4 years and six-month study of ayurveda and one year of residency program known as interneeship or housemanship. It is followed by post graduate study of ayurveda for three years leading to MD in ayurveda.

The word 'degree' has several meanings. In academics it is a stage in the vertical scale of education. A person who possesses graduate-level education is a graduate. A person who is engaged in the study beyond the graduation is a post-graduate. The growth of science & technology and spread of western-style education in India influenced the ayurvedic medical education.After the post-graduation, the person may engage in research leading to the award of doctor of philosophy or Ph.D. These degrees have to attest the depth of knowledge of the physician.

After five and half year course in ayurveda, some students prefer to pursue higher studies in ayurveda. Several topics of ayurveda like *śarira kriya, śarira rachana, dravyaguṇa, rasaśāstra, kāyacikitsa, śalya* are studied at the post-graduation level. After three-year study of ayurveda at post-graduate level, the doctors are awarded with MD (Ayu) degree. What is the difference in content of graduate and postgraduate courses of Ayurveda? In the three year MD course, the students again repeat topics they have already studied in the BAMS course, nothing more nothing new. This repetition is over in the first year. In the second year the students are asked to choose a topic of their interest. The students choose a topic and start writing a dissertation. Most of the chosen topics are either ridiculous or repeats of older topics. Thousands of students of *śalya* (general surgery) in the MD course have taken the sole topic 'hemorrhoids' and produced worthless theses. The quality of the postgraduate student is so poor and inadequate in knowledge that they cannot survive as successful ayurveda practitioners.

Several committees commissioned to oversee the ayurvedic education have contemplated to start postgraduate courses in ayurveda. Udupa committee (1958) was the first committee to emphasize on the postgraduate education in ayurveda. These committees have not visualized the content of the postgraduate courses. Thousands of the students join MD in ayurveda with a hope of better career. It is often pointed out that ayurveda is studied to not to practice but to teach! The CCIM has made it mandatory to have postgraduate degree in ayurveda to teach in ayurveda colleges for the appointments of lecturers made after 1989. More than half of the ayurveda colleges are in the private sector. Therefore, the postgraduate doctors of ayurveda find it easy to get a teaching position. Soon this is going to be saturated.

The government of India has appointed a Task Force to oversee the quality of education in AYUSH disciplines. The report of the Task Force is frank. It said that 'the general quality of AYUSH medical education remains very unsatisfactory. With some honorable exceptions, most AYUSH educational institutions do not provide quality medical education and the products of these institutions lack knowledge of the fundamentals of the system of medicine concerned. It was recognized that AYUSH education is just producing half-baked practitioners who are barely able to practice in the best traditions of their systems. More importantly, this lack of quality in the AYUSH practitioners is responsible for the decline in the quality of AYUSH health care delivery and is preventing AYUSH systems from playing an active role in the national health programmes'.

It recommended a new plan for coordination between various systems of medicine. 'It is essential that specialization should only be in classically recognized areas of the systems and not in artificially created areas merely on the analogy of specializations in allopathic medicine. Opportunities should also be created for the admission of ayurveda, yunani, siddha and homoeopathy graduates in system-neutral non-clinical post graduate medical courses like anesthesia, radiology, anatomy, physiology, optometry, hospital management etc. offered by allopathic medical colleges and other institutions instead of trying to create AYUSH versions of these specialties. It would also be necessary to start postgraduate diploma courses in specialties for AYUSH medical graduates at university level.

The report also speaks about breakdown of regulatory mechanism of ayurvedic education. 'The regulatory system created by the IMCC and HCC Acts has clearly been perverted by the regulatory Councils themselves in their single minded concentration on enabling more and more substandard new colleges to be set up. This has ensured that the elected seats on the Council have been effectively captured by non academic persons who run colleges or have a direct interest in the management of colleges. The Councils do not even go through the pretence of being concerned about academic standards or about the manner in which the medical colleges are being managed. The only issue, which concerns the Councils nowadays, is the opening of new colleges and, more importantly, the attendant activity of conducting inspections of the candidate colleges. The idealistic experiment of having autonomous regulatory Councils has most certainly broken down.'

Dominique Wujastyk, who was appointed as single-man committee to assess the status of ayurveda physician in the United Kingdom, observed that 'the training courses in ayurveda do not normally include modules on the history of the science, and the lack of general historical knowledge about Indian medicine amongst practitioners is shocking. Platitudes about ayurveda originating thousands of years B.C. are distressingly common'.Some international medical journals too have bitterly criticized the ayurvedic education in India. The Student Lancet from the United Kingdom opined that the ayurveda doctors trained in Indian colleges are neither fish nor fowl.

The greatest threat to AYUSH education in recent years has been the extraordinary growth of sub-standard private medical colleges. During the period 1996-2006, as many as 198 new colleges were set up, the vast majority being in the private sector. These colleges in general have little or no infrastructure in terms of the minimum standards prescribed; staffing levels are generally inadequate; and the quality of instruction is poor. Most of these newly opened colleges are churning out ill trained and barely educated AYUSH practitioners. The responsibility for this appalling situation rests entirely with the statutory Councils which actively colluded with the promoters to ensure that these colleges were set up in violation of the regulations issued by the Councils themselves with regard to minimum standards, staffing, infrastructure, etc.. To repair and regulate the education of ayurveda, the Task Force recommended setting up regional AYUSH universities. However, such structural changes are not going to improve the quality of education. Setting up of regional AYUSH universities will increase the tussles for power among the ayurvedaphysicians. Majority of ayurveda institutes have earned bad reputation because of caste politics.

To reflect the flavour of India, the CCIM has renamed the degrees awarded to the doctors. The BAMS course is known as *ayurvedacharya* and MD (Ayu) is known as *ayurveda vacaspati*. However, nobody uses this nomenclature in general practice. Several Indian arts are studied in the model devised by western education. However, the CCIM has not looked at the practicality and feasibility of the model adopted to teach ayurveda. The interdisciplinary and transdesciplinary studies are totally neglected in India. There are umpteen number of fields remain unstudied linking ayurveda to anthropology, sociology, history, linguistics, flora and psychology.

In the clinical practice of scientific medicine, different levels of drug protocols were developed. Qualified practitioners depending on their qualification in certain discipline prescribe certain formulations. An MBBS graduate is not authorized to prescribe, for instance, a latest anti-cancer drug like tomaxifen. Only a specialist with post graduate degree can do that. In ayurveda, the CCIM has not visualized different levels of drug prescription as in the case of scientific medicine. The graduates and postgraduates in ayurveda do not show any uniform protocols in drug prescription. The art of drug selection is as it was in medieval times. There is no restriction on any ayurvedic medicine to be prescribed by a graduate or post-graduate. This distinction between the graduate and postgraduate is mostly used to snob the society.

Few years ago, the government of Andhra Pradesh has introduced graduate and postgraduate courses in palmistry and astrology! There are professors, assistant professors and lecturers in these faculties. These academics have to be working on the issues of expediency of the astrology and palmistry; instead, they are striving as fortunetellers. Homoeopathy is losing popularity across the world but in India it is expanding as never before. The government of India does not want to disregard or ignore anybody or any discipline. Across the nation, new Vedic universities are being founded to rehabilitate impoverished Brahmins. Indians will not be surprised if the government sponsors institutes to teach and spread black magic, sorcery, talisman etc. All universities in India have been politicized. Appointment of chancellors and vice chancellors is a political decision based on the caste and other connections. Therefore, there is no hope of ayurvedic education getting any better.

The government of India has established several bodies, which often collide among themselves in administering alternative systems of medicine. There are Central Councils for research in ayurveda, siddha, homoeopathy, naturopathy and yoga. The government has created a big infrastructure for alternative systems of medicine and thus wants to appease all sections of the society. The activities of the councils and bodies are not properly evaluated.

Some diseases are earmarked in ayurveda as curable by praying to god (*daivavyapāsraya*); some are cured by the physician (*yuktivyapāśraya*) and some by the patient thyself (*satvāvajaya*). Thousands of temples and religious gurus across India promise good health and cure from incurables. The qualified ayurveda physicians of today wear aprons, use stethoscopes and pose like cosmopolitan medical doctors. Many young ayurveda graduates are sub-serving under modern doctors as assistants. Thus, the purpose of ayurvedic education is defeated. Therefore, reforms in ayurveda education are imminent and momentous. The report of the Task Force says 'the training should enable AYUSH doctors to handle patients and to diagnose conditions purely in terms of the accepted principles of the system concerned without unnecessarily taking recourse to the diagnostic techniques used in allopathic medicine.

In Europe and America, some universities started teaching ayurveda and other traditional medicines at graduate level. There is lot of criticism on these courses. David Colquhoun wrote in *Nature*, international weekly of journal of science, CAM courses offered in UK universities are anti-science. His article 'Science degrees without the science' also criticized the teaching of ayurveda under the heading of science. There are scores of such institutes offering science degrees sans science in the USA. This trend is an indication of corporatization of education.

Research in Ayurveda

There is a general opinion among the laity and the scholars alike that the government of India should encourage research in the field of ayurveda to modernize the system as well as to mend it to emerging health demands. Physicians and patients think research in ayurveda yields new medicines and therapies. The physicians of the modern medicine and empowered patients look at ayurveda for therapies for certain incurable diseases like HIV and cancer, for which the biomedicine is struggling to find therapies. Ayurveda physicians too wish to rise to the occasion. Indeed, they want to modernize ayurveda pharmacy and drug administration using new technology. The society always demands the best of both systems. Therefore, research and development are momentous and inevitable. However, what kind of research in ayurveda is going to help the system of medicine as well as the society?

Raw material for ayurvedic medicines are drawn from natural products available in nature. However, certain toxic substances like mercury, lead etc might enter the plant cycles and find their way into medicines. It was reported in several medical journals that many ayurveda medicines marketed across the world contain unacceptable levels of heavy metals. Ayurvedic medicines marketed within India escape rigorous testing and circumvent safety standards because of corruption and lax control over the field of pharmacy and clinical medicine. The ayurvedic medicines made out of innocuous herbs, as well as mineral formulations have to be tested for toxic constituents at unacceptable levels. Therefore, there is a demand for research on ayurveda formulations to render them safe for the general use. This research needs state-of-the-art laboratories, which can analyze the chemical constituents of ayurvedic formulations. Ayurveda scholars are not trained in such research to measure the levels of toxic ingredients in ayurvedic medicines. Ayurveda doctors trained in BAMS or MD (Ayu) study neither frontline biochemistry nor pharmacology. They are also not trained inrelevant instrumentation. Therefore, this research has to be carried out by the phyto-chemists and industrial chemists. Ayurveda physicians do not have avenues in this research.

Ayurveda medicines are older than the concepts of ayurveda.Ayurveda formulations may be effective in certain pathological conditions, because these medicines are empirical, time-tested and shown satisfactory results over a period of time. In rheumatoid arthritis, for instance, ayurveda prescribes castor oil and spices like pepper, long pepper and ginger. Similarly, the bark of the *arjuna* (Terminalia arjuna) tree is prescribed to prevent heart attacks. There are hundreds of such empirically tested herbs useful in varied clinical conditions. So, we need research to understand the drug action. The research to prove the worth of such ayurvedic products needs frontier level expertise in methodology. The knowledge of instrumentation, biochemistry, human physiology at higher level is necessary to interpret the drug action. Are ayurveda physicians capable of carrying such research? They cannot, because such study needs experts in biomedicine. The modern medical establishment supports techniques of isolating active principles from ayurvedic formulations. Indian Council for Medical Research and similar organizations in other countries are involved in such research. The ayurveda scholars are not able to carry out this work because they are not trained in either research methodology or modern chemistry.

The modern pharmaceutical industry looks at the traditional systems of medicine for treatment of diseases, which are incurable otherwise. It is presumed that traditional healers prescribed certain herbs containing some molecules effective in totally different pathological conditions but unaware of their uses. For example, the concept of blood pressure is unknown to ayurveda. The word *raktacapa* (blood pressure) is new to the vocabulary of ayurveda. However, the herb *sarpagandha*, Rauwolfia serpentina, is a centrally acting drug on hypertension. Ayurveda used it in sleeplessness, illusions and hallucinations, pains etc. The research has to be aimed at isolating molecules, which were not utilized by the traditional systems optimally. India has experience in modern scientific research of evaluating traditional medical herbs through laboratory testing. The Central Drug Research Institute in Lucknow is one such centre. The Central Council for Research in Ayurveda and Siddha (CCRAS) was established by the Government of India to exploit the herbal wealth of India in medicine. An ayurveda physician too cannot carry out this research because they are not trained in these methods. They are useful in literary research alone if they have good grounding in Sanskrit. CCRAS is indulged in the research into medicinal plants employing modern phytochemistry. The results acquired by the CCRAS are useful to the modern pharmaceutical industry. The CCRAS publishes its bi-monthly journal Medicinal and Aromatic Plants Abstracts (MAPA). Again the role of ayurveda graduates and post graduates in this arena is insignificant.

Ayurvedic literature alludes to hundreds of herbs. While many of these are clearly identified, there remains an important body of medicinal herbs whose identity is not certain. Research using botanical, historical, and literary sources can often clarify these matters, but this research depends essentially on knowledge of Sanskrit and vernacular languages of India along with sound knowledge of taxonomy. Therefore, the production of reliable information on ayurveda will be a task to be shared by Sanskritists, historians, linguists, anthropologists, botanists and doctors. Ayurveda physician alone can never carry out comprehensive research in ayurveda.

The interactions between some constituents in a pharmaceutical compound may be crucial to its modus operandi. This greatly complicates the testing of ayurvedic medicines. This kind of work too needs experts in physiology, biomedicine and phyto-chemistry. Considering all these protocols of research, the ayurveda physicians trained in B.A.M.S. or M.D. (Ayu) are not eligible or fit for research in ayurveda.

Unfortunately, the Central Council for Research in Ayurveda and Siddha (CCRAS) has carried out more *compilation* work rather than research work till now. After its existence of more than 40 years, the number of field units of CCRAS has come down to 29 from 89! The medicines produced by the CCRAS are not being extensively used in the ayurveda hospitals. Ayush-64 developed for malaria, Ayush-56 developed for diabetes are not popular among the physicians. The CCRAS has labored to produce an ayurvedic contraceptive, *Pippalyadi yoga*, which made headlines in newspapers two decades ago, is not available in the market. The physiologists do not believe that *pippalyadi* can effectively suppress ovulation as it was foreseen.

Ayurveda interprets the drug action as far as possible basing on the *rasa guṇa vīrya* and *vipāka* theory. *Rasa* is taste. Ayurveda presumes that there are six tastes in the nature: *madhura* (sweet), *amla* (sour), *lavaṇa* (salty), *kaṭu* (pungent), *tikta* (bitter) and *kaṣāya* (astringent). Each taste has its particular action on the body. *Guṇa* is property of a substance. There are ten pairs of properties like heavy and light, hot and cold. *Vīrya* is potency of a drug substance. *Vipāka* is post digestive action of a drug on the body. For example, the sweet, sour and salt tastes increase the quantity of feces; the pungent, bitter and astringent tastes decrease the quantity of excretory products. This appears to be a perfect theory to interpret the drug action. However, the action of several herbs does not fit into this framework. For instance, the plant Croton tiglium (*danti* or *nepāla*) is a strong laxative. The reasons are not understood basing on the *rasa* or *vipāka*. If the traits and end result of the drug substance is not tenable under the *rasa-guṇa-vīrya-vipāka* theory, *prabhāva* (special effect) is considered to be the reason. *Prabhāva* is an axiom. Some ayurveda physicians propose that research has to be oriented to find the *rasa guṇa vīrya* and *vipāka* of new drug substances that have recently entered the pharmacopoeia of ayurveda. Tomato, potato, chilly, groundnut, apple, custard apple, maize, carrot, sunflower and many more edibles have entered India and ayurveda pharmacopeia during the last five centuries. Ayurveda physicians are yet to decide on several properties of these new entrants. They do not put efforts in establishing the *rasa, guṇa, vīrya* of the new herbs that entered India after 15th century AD. On the other hand, they don't have an iota of interest to find out the nature of *prabhāva*. The research has to be directed towards the analysis of these traits in parameters attested by science.

Berkeley said, do not think, try. Indian ayurvedists spend more time in thinking rather than doing. Neither the methodology of ayurveda could lead us to scientific medicine, nor do the ayurvedic physicians digest the spirit of modern science to streamline system. The human societies have built the systems of medicine to serve the people. The purpose of any system of medicine is to serve the suffering humanity. The purpose of research is not to serve the system of medicine but the society.

Most of the ayurveda physicians feel that they have to *serve*ayurveda! They do not realize that serving people is more important than serving ayurveda. They take ayurveda as a religion that should be believed in.

Now, Indians are worried that the patent offices in other countries issue patents on India's indigenous knowhow to the foreign companies or persons. Ayurveda until now is considered as 'copyleft' domain; it suddenly turned to copyright. TKDL (Traditional Knowledge Digital Library) is an effort that brings together the Department of AYUSH, Council for Scientific and Industrial Research (CSIR) and the Ministry of Commerce and Industry. The data created will be available to the patent offices that issue patents. At the inauguration of TKDL in New-Delhi on 26 March 2002, the then Minister of Health and Family Welfare, C. P. Thakur emphasized that TKDL would play 'a crucial role not only in documenting our precious heritage in the area of traditional health-care systems, but also in preventing bio-piracy and un-scrupulous patenting of indigenous herbal medicinal formulations'. This was initiated to prevent issue of patents to once Indian discoveries. The ayurvedic formulations are recorded in English, French, German, Hindi, Japanese and Spanish. In future, it would be available in 20 foreign languages and all Indian languages.

Tracing the roots of ayurveda is a challenging task. The Dravidian roots of ayurveda have to be explored by an institution that is genuinely interested in the history of India. The establishment of Dravidian University in Kuppam,

Andhra Pradesh was a good beginning. The location Kuppam town was chosen because of its geographical proximity to the regions of the Dravidian languages. Kuppam is in the midst of Andhra Pradesh, Karnataka and Tamilnadu. It is also not far off from Kerala. When this university was founded in 1997, very few understood its importance. The university has responsibility in studying the Dravidian languages and Dravidian culture. If the scholars in this university neglect these topics, who else will do? Universities in Tamilnadu boast of Tamil pride and universities in Karnataka boast Kannada pride. Universities in Andhra Pradesh too occupy themselves with Telugu culture. Dravidian university is the only institution in South India that can shoulder the responsibility of research on Dravidian heritage. Unfortunately, this university too is obsessed with conventional courses like computer-software, teacher training, biotechnology etc. This is nothing but misemployment.

The Place of Sanskrit in Ayurvedic Studies

The Sanskrit grammar is taught to the students of ayurveda for 150 hours in the BAMS course. With this basic teaching, students are not able to read ayurveda treatises in original and understand them. Though much of ayurveda vocabulary in Sanskrit is intelligible to new students, their knowledge of Sanskrit is mostly passive. The question is, whether it is indispensable to know Sanskrit to gain good knowledge of ayurveda and to become good ayurveda physician?

There are many arguments for and against

Sanskrit in ayurvedic studies. If verses from the ancient scriptures are remembered, it is easy to remember the composition of ayurvedic formulations, signs and symptoms of diseases etc. A two gigabyte pen drive can remember important treatises of ayurveda and with a click required data is retrieved instantaneously. In this age of 'cheap memory', filling the brain with verses is not desirable. Instead, the brainpower can be used to focus on new areas of medicine. Many students of ayurveda detest study of ayurveda for this fact.

The knowledge cannot exist outside the sphere of language and language too cannot exist devoid of information and knowledge. Languages reflect the social eco-system where they evolved. There is no Esperanto, which can express every idea with ease. However, the modern European languages have gained rich and suitable vocabulary to express every nuance of modern life. If communism is studied without knowing German, Russian or Chinese, why not ayurveda without Sanskrit? The sole purpose of the language is to convey information and knowledge. Any language with enough vocabulary can do it. The student of ayurveda, who wants to practice clinical ayurveda, need not spend too much time in the study of Sanskrit.

Many erudite Sanskrit scholars point out that, ayurveda physicians in India are not properly versed in Sanskrit. The student of history of ayurveda needs to consult the manuscripts of the treatises to explore into history of ayurveda. So, the knowledge of Sanskrit is a prerequisite for them. Those, who study ayurveda as part of 'culture study', may have to acquire good command over Sanskrit. An ayurveda physician, who wants to practice traditional medicine, can study ayurveda in his or her mother tongue. Bertrand Russell titled one of his essays 'Useless Knowledge', wherein he says 'the utility of knowledge of Latin or classical Greek is questionable to the modern society'. Of course, he admits that some scholars may have to be occupied to possess such knowledge for future generations. We need some scholars like Priyavat Sarma, Dominique Wujastyk and Kenneth Zysk with expertise in the classical languages. We cannot expect all ayurveda physicians to be erudite Sanskritologists. Moreover, the medical vocabulary of Sanskrit is largely shared by the vernacular languages of India; therefore it is easy to grasp the meaning of medical terms in true spirit.

Sanskrit verses are uttered by the Brahmin priests in Hindu marriages or cremations. For many Brahmins this is their profession. But, Sanskrit is projected by the priest class as something mysterious. Whatever is said in Sanskrit is respectable, divine and it is a truth for many Indians. This mindset is perpetuated by the priest class since the Vedic times. It is difficult to find heretics among ayurveda physicians. Therefore no ayurveda physician in India reconsiders their opinion on the place of Sanskrit in ayurvedic studies.

Adam, a sanskritologist opined that classical writers of Sanskrit in ancient India were 'wasting their learning and their powers in weaving complicated alliterations, recompounding absurd and vicious fictions, and revolving in perpetual circles of metaphysical abstractions never ending still beginning.' In ayurveda too such alliterations and fantasies have overtaken the scientific thinking. The pedantic scholars are prone to commit mistakes in interpreting the concepts of ayurveda. If Caraka is living now, he would give up his ideas on humeral theory. Perhaps we are overcooking and misinterpreting the ideas and hypothesis to justify the ancient scholars. It's like interpreting a painting of Picasso. When Picasso draws an unsteady line, an art critic compares it with rhythm of life. Another art critic looks at wobbling line as the graph of share market. Though Picasso is silent, the interpreters take lead and create confusion. New breed of interpreters of concepts of ayurveda like Svoboda, Chopra, David Frawley and others are obsessed by overstretched imaginations and are distorting ayurveda.

Sheldon Pollack in his article, *Death of Sanskrit*, gives a realistic account of literary history of Sanskrit language. Sanskrit is neither a living language nor a dead language but a 'born dead' language! Ayurveda physicians and other scholars were more obsessed with language rather than science. Adherence to Sanskrit in documenting the inventions and discoveries in ayurveda has stunted the growth of scientific medicine in India. The entire ayurveda education is revolving around 10000 hymns of *Carakasamhita*. Ayurveda scholars think it is everything of medicine, the human mind can discover. Reinscription (copywriting older manuscripts) activity has engaged the ayurveda physicians more than original thinking and writing.

Raja Rammohan Roy, the pioneer of

renaissance in India, stated without any reservation 'the Sanskrit language, so difficult that almost a lifetime is necessary for its acquisition, is well known to have been for ages a lamentable check to the diffusion of knowledge, and the learning concealed under this almost impervious veil is far from sufficient to reward the labor of acquiring it'. Kabeer, the great Sufi reformer, likened Sanskrit to `the water of a well', and the language of the people to a 'running stream'. Shyam Rao thinks that 'the archaic nature of Sanskrit is evident in its vocabulary, which is highly synonymic, homonymic and hermaphroditic and its compounding nature. All these features render the language highly unsuited to communication and unfit for usage as a vernacular or language of science.' The phonetics and writing system of Sanskrit too is not congenial to modern India. The *devanagari* script, holy and revered form of writing, suffers from several defects. Writing in *devnagari* script is much slower compared to other scripts. Reading text in *devanagari* takes much longer time. It is commonly believed that the *devanagari* script has only 48 letters. However, if compound letters are considered, because the brain remembers the compound letters as separate patterns, the number of symbols in Sanskrit alphabet is more than five hundred. So illiteracy was ruling India, still is, because the language is unfriendly to knowledge and democratization of education was a far cry. Whenever, wherever Sanskrit dominated, illiteracy ruled the masses.

Patronization of Sanskrit by the kings in India has given a chance to the Brahmin community to traverse the land with ease. They have increased their field of activity. Their careers were bright. Today the Sanskrit studies are in deplorable condition. Once, the aspirants from non-Brahmin community were discouraged to study Sanskrit. Now the government of India encourages non-Brahmins to learn Sanskrit but it is very difficult to find students in spite of attractive scholarships, because the Sanskrit is the mouthpiece of Brahmin orthodoxy. There is no big difference between sanskritization and brahminization.

Thanks to the growth of modern linguistics, Sanskrit is no more a 'gods' language'. Nevertheless, Sanskrit is still considered a property of the Brahmin community in India. It is comparable to the Japanese in Japan. It is said that the Japanese don't appreciate if any foreigner speaks fluent Japanese. If any non-Japanese speaks fluent Japanese they become apprehensive and feel their land is being invaded. Similarly, if any non-brahmin is erudite in Sanskrit in India, that person is ignored by the majority of Sanskrit clergy. Fortunately, Sanskrit is just another classical language. It is a new sister to Latin and classical Greek, according to William Jones (1746 – 1794), the founder of the Asiatic Society. But the orthodox community in India does not remove the veil on Sanskrit. The role of Sanskrit in Hindu society is similar to that of Kallawaya language in South America. Both feed on the ignorance of the people.

The vocabulary of Sanskrit is rich and elaborate. It has potency to modernize the vernacular languages of India. It can be simplified in the model of Zamenhof's Esperanto. The simplified Sanskrit, perhaps with Roman alphabet, may become India's national language for all-round development. But the traditionalists don't let the Sanskrit to be useful for the future generations and casteless society. The Sanskrit has already rendered the vernacular languages of India unworthy of growth.

The chief trait of the Sanskrit knowledge is obscurantism. Today's ayurveda physicians create new verses in Sanskrit and propagate them as classical. In ayurveda education this practice is growing. Fortunately, a century ago the treatises of ayurveda were published. Now it is difficult to add new verses in the name of classical authors. But some new verses are entering in the textbooks of BAMS. This is not plagiarism but counter-plagiarism, i.e. ascribing modern thoughts to the ancient writers. Some obscurant scholars create some hymns sounding new concepts of medicine to create an opinion that they are already present in ancient treatises. They tambour about modernity of ayurvedic concepts. This happened in engineering and medicine. New Sanskrit verses were created after 1904 on building airplanes. These imaginary airplanes fly on urine of cow or elephant!

The image of ancient manuscript is divine to Hindus. It is considered authentic, respectable and beyond comprehension. Often ayurveda physicians boast that many manuscripts were missing and so the science of ayurveda is not able to compete with modern science. People think there are some missing links in ayurveda. Even if a new *samhita* is suddenly discovered, nothing new is going to be added. All the students of Ātreya tell the same story of ayurveda.

Is Ayurveda Scientific Medicine?

Many scholars and the laity take for granted that ayurveda is scientific medicine, which was popular in ancient India but lost its glory because of advent of Islam in the medieval period and western medicine in the colonial period. Ayurveda scholars say everything about health was perfect in the past. They oftentimes question why Hippocrates is the father of medicine, why not Caraka or Suśruta?

Hippocrates lived in 5th and 4th centuries BC in the island of Cos in ancient Greece. He was a member of the Guild of Aesculapidiae, which was established around 1250 BC in ancient Greece. The members of this Guild were devoted to the art of healing. They built temples to house the sick, and in each temple was a statue of Asclepius holding a staff with a snake coiled about it. This image of Caduceus has become the traditional symbol of medicine. Medical treatment was filled with belief and superstition. In such a system, Hippocrates was the first to theorize that all diseases are caused by physical factors. He did not believed in spirits or evil forces as etiological factors. Hippocrates was a visionary with clear mind and endowed with scientific spirit. He was the first to protect the privacy of the patients and recommend fair deal in medical practice. Hippocrates' Oath outlines the duties and responsibilities of physician in a capsule form. Although it has been rewritten several times, the basic tenets of the oath remain same. Hippocrates was the first to use the scientific method in medicine. He did not believe in the power of 'sin' in debilitating the body. The modern scientific medicine has sprung on the roots of Italian renaissance, which is the product of vision of ancient Hellenistic culture.

The magnum-opus treatises of ayurveda, almost contemporary to Hippocrates, are unanimous in believing in supernatural phenomena as causative factors for, if not all, many diseases. The epidemiology and etiology of several diseases in ayurveda are based on superstition and predetermined destiny. Strong belief in *karma,* role of sin in causing diseases played a vital role to stunt the growth of scientific medicine in India. The existing unjust social order (caste) and indolence of the intellectuals have unnerved the curiosity of people. Therefore, progress and creativity in sciences was a mirage in ancient India and so ayurveda did not favor the growth of scientific medicine.

Ayurveda itself is not scientific that fits the definition of science. Its theoretical premises were not translated into practice. It rather barred scientific thinking in India. Although the Indian philosophical systems ratify the knowledge verified by 'inference' as accurate, ayurveda could not absorb the growth of western medicine into its fold and get modernized. The modern science is nothing but the product of methodology using 'observation' and 'inference' described in the epistemology of ayurveda.

It was Hippocrates and ensuing scholars in the west, who founded modern school of thought in medicine. By all reasons, Hippocrates is the father of scientific medicine. Either Suśruta or Caraka cannot be considered as founders of scientific medicine, because the prejudices and approach to disease in ayurveda never lead us to scientific methodology. The historians of medicine classify ayurveda as empirico-rational medicine. There is a big gap between scientific medicine and empirico-rational medicine. The epistemological premises of the *nyaya* and *Vaiśeṣika darśanas*, on which the ideology of ayurveda is built, does not either reveal the true nature of the Nature. Ayurveda strongly believed that mind and soul (*ātma*) are different. It even considered brain as bone marrow.

Ayurveda is not a science. It is a cult and a culture. It has elaborate belief system. Its basic principles are a collection of contradictory hypotheses and speculations. The literature of ayurveda is filled with several internal contradictions, conflict of opinions, fantasies, blind beliefs, wild imaginations, speculations and premeditated ideas. The beliefs, practices and apprehensions with regard to health and disease have crystallized into ayurveda in ancient India. The scholars of ayurveda have forgotten the contributions of Buddhism to medicine.

In scientific medicine, growth of anatomy and physiology precede the development of pathology and medicine. In ayurveda, available little knowledge of anatomy and physiology is the consequence of practice of medicine! In other words, ayurveda pharmacopoeia and treatment flourished before the topics of anatomy, physiology and pathology were promulgated. Classical ayurveda texts do not entail the knowledge of human body in terms of its structure and function as essential before diagnosing the diseases. Hence, ayurveda is empirico-rational medicine. It is not scientific medicine in true spirit.

The word *science* too originally meant knowledge gained through experience, however, after the modern science has changed the lives and outlook on nature, the meaning of science has changed. The knowledge acquired using *scientific method* is science. Applied science is the knowledge applied in different disciplines like medicine and engineering. The scientific method employs five stages to collect knowledge – Problem or question, Observation, Hypothesis, Experimentation and Conclusion. There are innumerable problems in medicine/physiology. For instance Hansen's disease (leprosy) is caused by sin; *ātma* or soul exists; blood is transformed into muscle; bone marrow produces semen; increase of *vāta* decreases the sleep time etc. Suchhypotheses are found in the treatises of ayurveda. But no experiments were designed to prove the hypotheses. Therefore, majority of concepts of ayurveda are mere untested hypotheses.

Ayurveda derived its philosophical foundations from the *sankhya, Vaiśeṣika* and *nyāya darśanas*. These philosophical ideas do not help *transform* the nature. They are part of the history of philosophy. They are meant for understanding the *purpose* of the universe. The essence of these systems either does not allow a person to be rational. Blending materialism with idealism takes strange shapes in Indian philosophy. The scientific medicine has to be open-ended, but ayurveda is not. So it cannot be scientific. It insists on belief system and discourages questions.

The science comprehends the true nature of the time, space and matter. Its ability to look into nano-spaces and handling molecules gave us unsurpassed command to manipulate the biochemical pathways. This is made possible by unfettered creativity, unprejudiced approach and sincere teamwork. The science understood the chemistry of life as 'digital' in nature, i.e. the place and orientation of molecules in the genes is the deciding factor of all the characteristics in living beings. By altering the place of molecules, the desired traits can be achieved. But ayurveda thinks the nature is 'analog' in structure and function. Therefore, ayurveda tried to depend on physical traits (colour, weight, temperature etc) to understand the nature. It does not see discontinuity in the matter. While physics saw more empty space in the atom, ayurveda saw five elements, earth, water, fire, air and space as constituting elements. Therefore, the space element comprises only one fifth of the matter. These speculations are just history of physics and philosophy.

Integration of Ayurveda and Modern Medicine

India is a paradise for medical doctors. It's also a heaven for the practitioners of alternative systems of medicine. Medical pluralism is seen everywhere in India. In reality, inadequate state regulatory mechanisms are endangering the lives of the patients. The federal government and regional governments in different states support dispensaries of mainstream medicine and CAM systems. A patient is left to take his or her decision to choose the kind of treatment. Depending on the acuteness or severity of the disease, the patients choose the system of medicine. Often they seek advices from their friends and family members. Many rich and poor patients spend money for magic therapies in chronic conditions like HIV, cancer, alopecia, incurable skin conditions etc. Perhaps the government has to establish hospitals with CAM systems included as it was done in the erstwhile USSR. There is a debate going on for a long time on the issue of integration of modern medicine with ayurveda and/or other alternative therapies. Several official committees have studied this problem, but in practice the government is adhered to the status-quo arrangement. The main reason for this frozen situation is conflicting opinions from different groups of medical doctors in India. The debates and arguments go on and on, but the government is indecisive.

The word ‘integration’ is not yet defined satisfactorily. Ayurveda physician prescribing antibiotics cannot be considered as integration of ayurveda and scientific medicine. The physician of the mainstream medicine prescribing ayurveda medicine too cannot be the standard practice of integration. Appropriation of medical system to the needs of the people is integration.

An ideal system of biomedicine and clinical medicine would be teaching scientific medicine in the Indian languages initially at graduate level and introducing postgraduate courses in both western and alternatives systems. Thus a physician of ayurveda or yunani will have a basic knowledge of biomedicine, therefore the fruits of CAM systems will reach the patient.

The specialists in biomedicine and policy makers at the Medical Council of India are still wary of the proposal to teach medicine in vernacular languages of India. Until and unless we study science and technology in our languages, the creativity is a far cry. The topics of health and medicine are in the 'concurrent' list of the Indian constitution. Therefore, the central and state governments have their share of duties and responsibilities in the health sector. The rights and privileges of the practitioners are taken care by the respective state/regional governments. A state government may sanction the right of prescribing modern medicines (antibiotics and painkillers) to ayurveda doctor to treat patients in critical conditions. In several states, th law prohibits ayurveda physicians from prescribing modern medicines. This will obviate the removal of the word 'Surgery' from 'Bachelor of Ayurvedic Medicine and Surgery', because without modern antibiotics and anesthetics surgery is impractical and illegal.

Because of special relationship of India with the United Kingdom, many ayurveda physicians have moved to Britain to practice ayurveda. The British government has appointed a committee to oversee the issues and visualize a plan to authenticate the practice of ayurveda in Britain. Dominique Wujastyk, a well known Sanskrit scholar and historian of ayurveda has compiled a thought-provoking report. This report tried to evaluate a plan licensing system for ayurveda physicians in Britain. Inter alie the report stated that 'critics of the college-based ayurvedic education, which aims to teach a mixture of ayurveda and basic medical science, argue that these colleges produce students who are neither fish nor fowl: they are not trained thoroughly in either ayurveda or biomedical science. Standards in Sanskrit language are very poor; teaching is in English or the local state language. The educational situation in India is complicated by the fact that training in ayurvedic medicine is sometimes seen as an option for students who fail entry requirements for biomedical medical school but who still want a profession in medicine.

'In pre-colonial times, education in ayurveda was principally conducted in traditional Sanskrit schools in which students started very young (10 or less), and were grounded for over 12 years in the Sanskrit language and in the medical literature. Apprenticeship to a practicing physician was also essential. Unlike China, pre-modern India did not develop a system of medical licensing, and the right to practice, as well as professional success, was a function of good reputation, training by a famous teacher, and sometimes court patronage.

Nobody could summarize better than Dominique Wujastyk on the quality of new age ayurveda publications. 'There has been an explosion in the publication of popular works promoting ayurveda as a new therapy. All these books are written by authors who are primarily interested in promoting Ayurvedic therapy in practice. But these authors may not have either an awareness of historical issues bearing on ayurveda, or any linguistic abilities in Sanskrit. They may have a strong vested interest in increasing their client base.

The committee examined the topics of patient satisfaction, the role of the therapist, the placebo effect, the evidence for efficacy and safety, statutory- and self-regulation, professional training and education of practitioners, research and development in CAM (including methodology and funding), public information dissemination, and CAM health-care delivery. The report divided CAM therapies into three large groups. While Homeopathy enters the group I, ayurveda entered into group 3. In the aftermath of the publication, the Indian Government went as far as to send a delegation of senior ayurvedic practitioners to the House of Lords to meet Lord Walton and discuss the Group 3 classification given to their practice! It is not worried about other aspects of ayurvedic education explained in the report.

Institutional Research in the History of Ayurveda

Ayurveda colleges in India teach *ayurvedaitihas* (history of ayurveda) to the undergraduate students of ayurveda for fifty hours in the first year of course. The teachers of *ayurvedaitihas* are inclined to impart mythology of ayurveda rather than the secular history of medicine. Moreover, ayurveda colleges do not consider this subject as one of the serious topics of ayurveda. The post-graduate centers of ayurveda too do not emphasize much on the realistic history of Indian medicine. Majority of ayurveda students are interested in clinical aspects of ayurveda. Therefore, the net result of the researches in the history of medicine conducted in the ayurveda institutes across the country is insignificant.

The Indian Institute of History of Medicine with its headquarters in Hyderabad, Andhra Pradesh, is an important institution providing useful information to the scholars interested in the history of medicine. This institute is now administered by the Central Council for Research in Ayurveda and Siddha (CCRAS). This was founded in 1950s on recommendation by Henri Sigerest, a historian of medicine with worldwide reputation. He visited India on a request from the Bhore committee, constituted to examine the nature of medical education in India by the then British government. This institute maintains a good library and subscribes to important journals of history of medicine from across the world. There is a good collection of antiques too. It publishes a quarterly *Bulletin of Indian Institute of History of Medicine*. The library and museum of this institute need a revamp.

Several post-graduate centers of ayurveda in India *viz.* Banaras Hindu University (Varanasi, Uttar Pradesh), Gujarat Ayurved University (Jamnagar, Gujarat), and National Institute of Ayurveda (Jaipur, Rajasthan) etc. assign the students and researchers different topics of history of ayurveda in the departments of Basic Principles. Some of these dissertations produced in these institutes deal with the history of medicine in India. The quality and originality of these researches is questionable. Many of the ideas in these researches are naïve and plagiaristic.

Few scholars of Ancient Indian History from some universities in India are focusing on the history of ayurveda. The Indian History Congress is yet to concentrate on the history of ayurveda. The regional History Congresses in India are now accepting papers on the history of ayurveda. The number of these papers so far is very small. Indian History Congress has once remembered Dwarakanath, a renowned ayurveda scholar and historian, in one its sessions 'Shaping of Indian Sciences 1940-80'.

The well known writings of foreign scholars on history of ayurveda are Dominik Wujastyk of Great Britain, Muelenbeld of Netherlands, Kenneth Zysk of Denmark are few to mention. Unfortunately these names are not popular among the ayurveda teachers in India. There are hundreds of professors of ayurveda in ayurveda colleges carrying their lives without updating their knowledge but spending their time in petty college politics. Most of the books written by the teachers of ayurveda are useful only to the students to pass in the BAMS examinations but not useful to make advances in science.

Theory and Practice of Ayurveda

From 19th century AD onwards, ayurveda started facing wider global audience. It was the age of reason and scientific medicine in Europe.

Progress in biological and physical sciences dispelled old beliefs in medicine. The physicians in India were exposed to science. Consequently, the ambiguities in the practice of ayurveda are caught the attention of Europeans. Once the influence of scientific medicine made a dent on ayurveda, scholars were divided on the issue of interpretation of principles of ayurveda and integrating these two systems. In the 20th century, ayurveda physicians were stumbled by the unhindered progress of scientific medicine.

In India, it is very difficult to find ayurveda physicians who try to understand and reconcile differences between allopathic medicine, as it is known in India, and ayurveda system of medicine. Svoboda, Deepak Chopra, David Frawley and others assert that ayurveda is a product of Indian soil and it is going to be a revolution in health care industry. They reinterpret concepts of ayurveda as eternal principles. David Frawley tries to convince the reader about greatness of Vedic ideas. Reading his books makes you more sick and esoteric. He says ayurveda is vegetarian medicine!

Deepak Chopra was exposed to ayurveda in early 80s and worked with Maharishi Mahesh Yogi. Chopra believes in the power of ayurveda to trigger miraculous healing in chronic diseases. The writings of Chopra do not appeal to scholars. They aim at gullible patients and non-serious self-styled philosophers. Svoboda studied BAMS in India in 70s and writes prolifically on ayurveda. Language is the only mesmerizing part of the writings of Svoboda. After closing the book, you do not remember anything worth. These writers strongly believe in the dogma of ayurveda and they try to rationalize it. They have good coverage in world media, and their books are designed attractively to allure innocent patients and curious readers. These books are meant for eulogizing tradition, whether it is rational or irrational. Other scholars like Kenneth Zysk, Dominik Wujastyk, and Muelenbeld are interested in tracing real history of ayurveda. They learned Sanskrit and studied ayurveda not to treat patients. Their writings are going to influence the future of history of medicine.

Close examination of the treatises convey that *tridoṣas* are considered 'material' in nature by ancient ayurvedists. However, Svoboda thinks *tridhoshas* are *non-material* substances guiding the bodily functions. Majority of ayurveda physicians of India today are not bothered to know whether *tridoṣas* are tangible or intangible substances. Some even argue.. is electricity or magnetism visible? Although electricity and magnetism are not visible to the naked eye, these forces are harnessed and measured. But *tridoṣas* are the products of imagination so they cannot be harnessed. The three humors, *vāta, pitta* and *kapha*, are further classified into five categories each. The students of ayurveda rote-learn Sanskrit verses describing five divisions of *vāta, pitta* and *kapha* regarding their locations and functions. However, this knowledge is never applied in practice.

Vireśvara, a bright student of Vihārilāl Miśra in the 17th Century AD in Rajasthan, refused humoral theory and proposed a new theory of pathology. He says 'the greatest authorities define disease as identical to an inequality in the humours. And yet, in other places they say that the humours may naturally exist in different quantities, without causing illness, such as when phlegm naturally predominates at the start of the day, or after a meal. This is not to say that one is always ill after a meal. And so the central doctrine that humoral inequality is identical with disease must be wrong'. The argument he started was unheeded. Today's ayurveda scholars are not interested in those unpublished ancient and medieval texts except the Big Three!

Syncretism has become a way of thinking among ayurveda physicians. Split-mind approach of ayurveda scholars has not helped ayurveda to transform into scientific medicine. Ayurveda physicians still think humeral theory is sufficient to explain pathology of all diseases. They never ever bothered to measure and to objectivise subjective narration. Vast gulf between theory and practice of ayurveda is proved by several elements. The description of *marma* (vital) points over human body is essential for the students of ayurveda in anatomy. Once anatomy subject is over in BAMS course, the student never encounters an occasion to use this knowledge clinically. Either *kāyacikitsa* or *śalyaśalākya* subjects do not use this knowledge for treatment. This part of the knowledge has become only a theoretical entity without practical utility whatsoever.

The students of physiology (*śarirakriya*) come across several such useless ballasts, useful only to get good marks in university examinations.

The concept of *shatcakra* (six wheels) in the spine, usually dealt in *tantric* literature, is taught to the students of ayurveda. It is said that the presence of so-called *kundalini* power in dormant state in the base (*muladhara cakra*) of the spine can be awakened by meditation and penance. If this power rises to *svadhishtana* (base of pudenda) and successively through the *manipura* (umbilicus), *anahata* (heart), *visuddha* (throat) and *ajna* (between the eyes in the head), different supernatural powers can be acquired! This knowledge does not have clinical application in the practice of ayurveda. The *ojas* (quintessence of seven *dhātus*), ayurveda asserts, is essential to understand the immunity. The description suggests that *ojas* is a tangible substance. It has color, smell and volume. New scholars, who are not able to show this tangible substance, even after the advent of modern anatomy, emphasize that *ojas* is not visible but it *is* present.

Just ten percent of herbs described in ayurveda make up ninety percent of ayurvedic pharmaceutical products. Twenty herbs, vastly used in ayurveda, can be found in almost all ayurvedic formulations. Most prominent among them are *haritaki* (Terminalia chebula), *vibhitaki* (Terminalia bellerica), *āmalaki* (Phyllanthus emblica), *ardrak* (Zinziber officiale), *pippali* (Piper longum), *marica* (Piper nigrum), *yaṣṭimadhu* (Glycyrrhiza glabra), hing (Ferula asafoetida), *vaca* (Acorus calamus), *tila* (Sesamum indicum), laśuna (Allium sativum), aśvagandha (Withania somnifera), haridra (Curcuma longa), bilva (Aegle marmelos) etc. These herbs have to be reevaluated for their quality and ingredients as each herb will have wide variation of ingredients depending on various climatic conditions. In Kerala, more than 90 varieties of black pepper are identified!

Media is reporting adversely on fly-by-night ayurveda massage centers in Kerala, which are attracting scores of healthy foreign tourists every day. The Hindu reported under a rubric Hawkers of Malady, 'centers offering ayurvedic cures and rejuvenation therapies mushroom on the beaches of the city (Tiruvanantapuram) during tourist season. Ill-equipped and inept, these centers pose a threat to tourist's health.' There is a need for standardization and accreditation of these centers. Many of the so-called *pancakarma* centers or Kerala *pancakarma* centers apply preparatory methods like oil massage and say this is *pancakarma*.

The evolution of treatment protocol should be a prime concern of the academic institutes of ayurveda. If ayurveda hospital wants to be honest to its methodology in diagnosis and treatment, a patient has to be examined for *Prakṛti* (constitution), the signs and symptoms of the disease as explained in the treatises. The differential diagnosis has to be made without the help of modern diagnostic techniques. Employing modern diagnostic methods like X-ray or Magnetic Resonance Imaging do not add any additional information to the disease picture narrated in ayurveda, because *tridoṣas* or their vitiation is not seen by the eyes. Ayurveda treatises depend more on symptoms rather than on signs of diseases. Symptoms are the feelings of the patient while the signs are the findings of the physicians without modern diagnostics. No institute is working in this direction. However, recent syncretic works are encouraging ayurveda physician to employ modern diagnostic technology in diagnosis. Although the state does not prohibit the ayurveda physicians from depending on the modern diagnostic methods, this practice is an indication of dichotomy between the theory and practice of ayurveda. A survey conducted suggested that 90 percent of the ayurveda physicians in India try to diagnose the diseases according to scientific medicine. No treatise of ayurveda talks of kidneys as blood-filtering organs and therefore producing urine. Measuring blood pressure and using stethoscope to listen to the heart sounds were never a diagnostic method in ayurveda. How to accommodate the know-how of ayurveda into realistic knowledge of western medicine? The scholars and students, therefore, develop split-mind approach. There are two main reasons for this anti-science behavior; a belief instilled into the minds of ayurveda scholars that it is complete science and syncretism as a way of justifying it. An ideal ayurveda physician visualizes diagnosis without being distracted by the syncretism. However, the question is how far this diagnosis is amenable to treatment? The treatment protocol too has to be standardized, as several ayurveda treatises often recommend contradictory treatments. The Ayurveda Pharmacopoeia Committee of India compiled most of the ayurveda pharmaceutical preparations and it is on the way to evolve a uniform protocol in the ayurveda treatment. The students of ayurveda have to be sensitized to this evolution and changing protocols of treatment.

The scope of ayurveda and other CAM systems in public health is totally misunderstood. It is apt to compare ayurveda to 'health manual'. If we buy a television set or any electrical/electronic gadget, we get a manual along with it. The manual helps you to fix it and use. It can also guide you to troubleshoot. However, major repairs are fixed only by a technician. The manual is not intended to explain total structure and function of the gadget. It doesn't teach you the entire mechanism of electronics inside. Similarly, the whole literature of ayurveda is a 'health manual' to enjoy the life. It never bothers to explore the structure and function (anatomy and physiology) of the human body. It suggests you what to eat, what not to eat, when to eat and when not to eat. But don't ask, why? So, we find strange theories in the concepts in ayurveda on anatomy, physiology, etiology and patho-physiology. Basing on this analogy, ayurveda can never explain the meaning of life or critical human physiological processes. It is also naïve to think that ayurveda starts where modern medicine ends.

In India today, majority of young ayurveda practitioners are serving in the western medical hospitals as physician assistants. Those who work in the government and private ayurveda colleges and hospitals too do not practice ayurveda. The number of doctors practicing ayurveda is discouragingly less. The ayurveda pharmaceutical companies too depend on 'over the counter sales' and allopathic doctors for their market. Unethical practices are on the rise. The state does not supervise who is practicing ayurveda and whether they are qualified. As stated in the foreword, pharmacists, meditations teachers, botanists, saffron-clad gurus etc practice ayurveda. The media focuses on mostly charlatans and dollar-hungry pseudo scholars. As long as institutionally qualified ayurveda physicians live in their cocoons the situation is not going to change.

Ayurveda treatment, veritably, does not depend on elaborate laboratory investigations because the classical texts of ayurveda emphasize more on symptoms rather than signs of diseases. The symptoms are narrated by the patient and signs are identified by the physician without depending on the laboratory data. There is no uniform opinion among the ayurveda physicians on using the laboratory data in therapy. Ayurveda consultants do not hesitate asking for Magnetic Resonance Imaging from the patients although they do not know basics of reading MRI films.

Nanjanagud is a small town in Mysore district of Karnataka state. This small town is known for Ayurvedic medicines with good quality since a long time. Dr B.V. Pandit, who established Sadvaidyasala in the previous century, is well known across the region. An ayurvedic tooth powder produced from Nanjangud is equally famous before the toothpastes could penetrate villages and towns in south India.

Some Traditional Centers of Healing

By virtue of some accidental discoveries and decentralized professionalism of medical practice in India, some families acquired fame as effective healing centers for some earmarked diseases. Some of these centers are popular for a long time. New centers of medical cults are coming up from time to time.

Puttur, a small town in south Andhra Pradesh, is located at a distance of 30 k.m. from the busiest Hindu pilgrim town of Tirupati. *Putturu kattu* (Bandage of Puttur) has little changed over 125 years of its popularity. The 'Puttur bandage' of Surapuraju Subba Raju family is highly acclaimed by the people not only in Andhra Pradesh but also from far off places in Tamilnadu and Karnataka. Eggs of hen, grinded leaves of Cassia tora (*cakramarda*) are made to a paste in an oil base, applied on the skin at the site of bone fractures, and tied in layers of cloth for immobilization. In spite of new orthopedic hospitals across the region, the rush to Putturu bone-setting hospital has not come down. The tradition believes that the leaves of *cakramarda* heal the bone better than any other medicine. In fact, the paste applied does not at all influence the process of bone healing. Immobilization is the key in bone healing. The positive aspect of this hospital is that service in this hospital is gratis. However, patients may donate money, as they like. Hence, it is very popular in this region, especially among poor sections of the society.

There are tens of places across India, famed as healing centre of 'Bells palsy' (facial paralysis) and general paralysis. Until 1980s, the people of south India tried to call a person known as Pamula Narasaiah over telephone to get rid of snake poison by his 'magic chant'. Impressed by his service, then British government has provided him with a job as Assistant Station Master in his native place in Andhra region to serve people. Many victims of snakebite used to visit him and those who cannot because of distance, can contact him over a toll free telephone.

Another important fad in healing traditions of India is Fish medicine popularized by Bathini Goud brothers of Hyderabad, the capital of Telangana. For the past one hundred and fifty years, this family has earned reputation as healers of bronchial asthma, by administering medicine through a small Murrel fish. Healer pushes small fish loaded with some yellow paste of medicine, into patient's throat. This medicine has to be taken consecutively for three years on a specified day. The vegetarians can take the medicine with jaggery instead of fish. Medicine, that is administered through a fish is examined by this author and found that it contains turmeric, jaggery, pepper and some dough as a ground substance. The medicine is administered in *mrigasira karti nakshatra* (Orionis) in the month of June before the onset of monsoon. 'Fish medicine' is an example of the decentralization of ayurveda in ancient India.

Kerala is known for several such healing techniques. There is one exclusive ayurveda hospital to treat patients of snakebites. Parassinikadavu Ayurvedic Hospital near Kannur in Kerala is known for treating snakebites. Their website says that they have saved ten million victims! A visit to the hospital will clarify that they have stopped depending on herbal extracts in treating victims of poisonous snake attacks. Ankola oil of Karnataka is known to cure paralysis. Ankola is a place name. Coimbatore in Tamilnadu was also known for orthopedic treatment to straighten the club foot. In this treatment an herbal potion was used to soften the bone.

There are innumerable techniques used in these healing homes. These techniques are not available in the BAMS courses. A wide variety of healing and folklore practices have gained fame under the category of ayurveda.

The Problem of Siddha

It is not 'the problem of siddha' but the presence of siddha medicine as a problem for ayurveda. The popularity of siddha medicine in south India not only makes a dent on ayurveda but also creates a big vacuum in ayurvedic market of South India. Although siddha medicine barrowed much of its philosophy and concepts from ayurveda and other Asian counterparts, it does not takes ayurveda as its past. Tamil culture declines to accept the authority of Sanskrit. The Dravidian movement in Tamilnadu in 1950s and 60s has virtually weakened the Brahmin domination on the Tamil society. This movement has helped the Tamil people to find their roots and pride.

Sanskrit and ayurveda are not going to gain ground in Tamilnadu. The Dravidian movement too has not crossed the borders of Tamilnadu. The Justice party, a political party originated to oppose Brahmin domination in pre-independence politics in the British Raj, was gradually waned.

Kerala has travelled the other way. The cultural movement of Narayana Guru, an Ezhava by caste, has advanced the understanding of the people regarding Brahmanism. The oppressed were allowed to enter into Hindu temples. Kerala was the first state in India to elect a communist government through ballot. Social reforms in Kerala have helped the society in several ways. However, siddha medicine is not popular in Kerala. The Dravidian movement was not popular in Karnataka. The influence of Jainism and *virasaiva* movement on ayurveda physicians in Karnataka is obvious. The popularity of the *Basavarājiya* is an attestation to this fact.

The Indian Medical Practitioners' Cooperative Stores (IMPCOPS) in Chennai is a prestigious and well-organized pharmaceutical unit in cooperative sector manufacturing ayurveda and siddha medicines since 1949. In quality and price, the products of Impcops are preferable to any other pharmacompany of ayurveda. There are thousands of practicing physicians from siddha and ayurveda fields that run the company. The management of Impcops is not much interested in ayurveda wing. Impcops tries to push more siddha medicines than ayurveda medicines. Ayurveda share holders of the company, spread over entire south India, are not able to get organized to have their own cooperative unit, because ayurveda physicians are allured by multinational companies and not interested in supporting medicines manufactured by Impcops in cooperative sector.

The government of Tamilnadu does not sponsor ayurveda education but runs several siddha educational institutes under the Dr MGR Medical University, Chennai. The official language in siddha colleges is not Sanskrit but Tamil. All existing ayurveda colleges in Tamil Nadu are in private sector. However, state Medical University does examinations and certification. Only recently an ayurvedic college was opened by the Government of Tamilnadu in Nagarcoil. In near future, there is no scope for ayurveda to flourish in the state of Tamilnadu.

Siddha physicians are more self-confident than ayurveda physicians because they don't have the problem of linguistic obscurantism. They love their language and do not take Sanskrit as authentic or divine. Siddha physicians may be wrong in their opinion that siddha medicine was not influenced by ayurveda. However, it is a blessing that Sanskrit is not going to bother them.

Reorganizing Ayurveda

Ayurveda is one of several sectors lacking in leadership and vision. The political leaders of India in the 20th century were immersed in agitations for securing independence and least bothered about social and economic reconstruction in independent India. The physicians too have to take equal responsibility for confusing the politicians. However, professors of ayurveda do not think they are in trouble. They are in a state of euphoria. They do not realize their duties and responsibilities. Majority of bureaucrats heading ayurveda establishments in India too are unscholarly, myopic and inherently feudalistic. Reorganizing this field is one of the difficult tasks India is facing. We need a roadmap for revamping ayurveda in India.

Ayurveda is one of the least organized professional groups in India. One can find hundreds of associations, conflicting opinions on teaching, treatment and research and varying levels of state patronage in different parts of the nation. Policy makers and planners are not inclined to understand internal problems of this discipline.

Scientific medicine is rational and technology savvy. It may not be cost effective but goal specific and result oriented. The principles of allopathy are instantly applicable and universally replicable. Charles Leslie, a medical anthropologist, opines that scientific medicine is not so scientific in application, i.e. it is in access to only a few, who can afford. In contrast, ayurveda has traits to become truly a people's medicine, but it is limping in the process of institutionalization. Modern medicine is an essential state service but ayurveda is viewed as non-essential service. Ayurveda scholars often complain that budget allotted to ayurveda is trivial, but they do not have plans to spend huge budget.

Preventive potential of ayurveda is more than its curative potential. It is powerless in fighting against tropical and communicable diseases. Today most of the state ayurveda dispensaries are located in rural areas, where people need protection against communicable diseases and epidemics. Urban places host several private ayurveda clinics attracting affluent patients. Most of these hospitals are not properly supervised by the state. The governmental registry of ayurveda doctors does not look into the way of practice of registered ayurveda physicians. Without registration, too one can practice ayurveda in India! So lax is the law.

The government of India is trying to mainstream CAM systems and encouraging referrals among different systems of medicine. This is an encouraging sign towards integration. However, this is not sufficient until some radical changes are made in functioning of CCIM, syllabus of BAMS, compelling ayurveda physicians to stick to their methods and stringent drug control. Preventing exploitation of ayurveda by quacks and development of various levels of treatment protocol are needs of the day.

Ayurveda scholars in different parts of India have ignored the potential of vernacular languages in growth of medicine. Sanskrit language has led ayurvedic society into snobbery. The English language is now displacing Sanskrit. Sanskrit and English have pushed vernacular languages of India into a moribund state. In medieval Europe, growth of science and technology has been hastened not by Latin but by modern languages (English, French, German etc.) of Europe. Today India needs an integrated approach and clear language policy in medical education. Physicians in India cannot imagine that modern medicine could be studied in vernacular languages. Medicine is studied in English in Britain, the USA and other English speaking countries, in French in France, in German in Germany, in Dutch in Netherlands, in Italian in Italy, in Russian in Russia, in Chinese in China, in Japanese in Japan, even in Persian in Iran, but medicine is studied in English in India! India had inherited this baggage. In addition, it has become a big health hazard. Many universities in India have implemented English medium in ayurveda colleges too. Teaching ayurveda in English language is not going to modernize it. Innocence and snobbishness are two impediments that affect progress of ayurveda.

Indian government often proposes structural change in the name of reforms. Obviously, structural changes cannot bring about functional efficiency. Change at individual level is starting point for reform. Unless and until the primary and secondary education is revamped, attitudinal change would not happen. Failure of education is the biggest cause of all this mess in medicine. We have a habit of pointing to the British as a pretext for failures even after seven decades of independence. The personnel of the Indian Administrative Service, who run most of the departments of ayurveda, could not rudder boat of ayurveda. Caprice actions of ayurveda bureaucracy have created umpteen numbers of problems to CAM systems.

Poor communications and transport facilities, ignoring vernacular languages too played a vital role in keeping ayurveda in suspended animation in medieval India. The sphere of ayurveda is mostly filled with half-baked ayurvedic scholars, who are self-centered and caste-conscious. Their energy and skills are not doing enough to Indian health sector. Majority of ayurvedic physicians in India are not aware of the place of ayurveda in healthcare. Ayurveda physicians in India do not appreciate unbiased study of history of ayurveda by western scholars. Prejudiced opinions and indolence ultimately led the discipline of ayurveda into a state of oblivion. They are elated by titles given by universities like professor, principal, rector, dean, director etc. Until and unless they come out of their 'paradise', nobody can save them from impending doom. A mediocre ayurveda physician believes in ayurveda gods and *pancamahābhuta* and *tridoṣa* concepts as valid explanations to drug action. He depends on modern diagnostics to examine the patient and yet thinks ayurveda is divine. They do not take pains to reconcile the philosophical gaps between modern and ayurveda disciplines. The government too is not looking at prospects of integration of ayurveda with modern medicine for maximum benefit to health care industry.

Without putting in hard work ayurveda physicians cannot do justice to their duty. Their academic acumen can be measured by their patronizing journals of ayurveda. There are thousands of medical journals published across the world periodically. For instance, Nature, an interdisciplinary magazine started in 1869 from Britain, is published every week with more than 53,000 paid subscriptions. Lancet, another important medical journal has diversified into several specialized journals with thousands of copies each. The New England Journal of Medicine, from the US has a circulation of 200,000 every week! In India, there are around 20,000 ayurveda teaching faculty but there are less than ten ayurveda journals periodically published and each one subscribed by just one or two hundred doctors. The quality of these journals too is very low. Some pharmaceutical companied publish few journals to advertise their products with lot of cooked up data.

Although there are no 'if's in history, it is interesting to imagine the state of ayurveda, if the British have not colonized India. What would be the state of ayurveda if India had escaped colonization like Japan? The basic principles of ayurveda, the *pancabhuta* theory, the *saptadhātu* theory etc. obviously do not lead physician of ayurveda towards scientific medicine. Institutionalization of ayurveda would be delayed by another century. If Macaulay system of education was pushed on India in 1830s, at that time there were Hindu kingdoms in India (Mysore etc.), where Indians could go with their plan of education, but that has not happened. Anatomy and physiology are key subjects for progress of scientific medicine. Any progress in physiology is destined to yield good results in medicine.

Many scholars have tried to modernize ayurveda. Several articles were written in different journals in vernacular languages between 1900 and 1950. These articles tried to teach chemistry to alchemists and botany to herbalists. Today, ayurveda colleges continue with ambiguous syllabus and nebulous ideas on their role in health care industry. The sanctification of ayurveda and syncretism between allopathy and ayurveda are two forces that are propelling ayurveda into future. This is highly distressing.

The government of India may look into the possibility of integrating the scientific medicine with CAM systems of medicine and teach in national languages of India to discourage brain drain to other countries and appropriate the knowledge of medicine to suit the needs of India.

This will also heighten the prestige of ayurveda physician in India. It is time to learn from experiences of other countries like China and Russia, where traditional systems of healing were incorporated into mainstream medicine and taught in local language. Undergraduate degree of BAMS is not properly serving health needs of India. Majority of BAMS graduates serve in modern nursing homes as 'less than a doctor and more than a nurse'. The future of students, who join ayurvedic courses, is being tarnished forever. Bertrand Russell has put it 'the human being has to be inspired by love and guided by knowledge'. This is what exactly lacking in the land of Buddha.

Yoga and Ayurveda

Yoga is more popular and acceptable than ayurveda outside India. Ayurveda prescribes medication but yoga is a drugless approach to health. Yoga is non-invasive. Yoga is a doctrine teaching the way of liberating soul (*ātma*) from this mundane world. On the contrary, ayurveda strives to enhance lifespan and help enjoy life. Both are equally misused, misinterpreted and are commoditized.

The word yoga comes from Sanskrit word *yugma* (join). Yoga is meant for salvation. Like ayurveda, yoga too is *Aṣṭānga* (eight-branched); *yama* (restraint), *niyama* (injunction), *āsana* (posture), *prāṇāyāma* (regulation of breathing), *pratyāhāra* (withdrawal of mental faculties), *dhāraṇa* (concentration), *dhyāna* (meditation) and *samādhi* (unification/immobile contemplation of mind). Patanjali reformed the way of yoga from *haṭhayōga* to *rājayōga*, from physical to psycho-corporeal.

It is surprising that modern yoga is used to stay fit. There are many theories expounding the mode of efficacy of yoga in certain diseases. Empirically yoga helps reduce arthritis, sleeplessness, anxiety etc. How does it work? I found the answer for this question in Japan! In 1994-95, I was studying a sino-japanese technique called 'yumeiho' therapy in the Institute of Preventive Medicine in Tokyo. Dr Masayuki, the founder of the institute, once met a scholar from Shaolin temple in China, who taught him a secret in human physiology. We suppose that body weight is borne by two legs equally. However, the body weight of bipedal human being is not born by two legs equally. Instead, it is shared disproportionately leading to some tilt in pelvis and therefore spine slightly bends to either side. The bent of spine (mild kyphosis, scoliosis, lordosis etc) gives unequal pressure over the nerve roots (ramii) leading to discomfort and several diseases. The Yumeiho therapy is aimed at correcting the curvature of spine and making it erect and symmetrical. One hundred plus techniques are used to press-knead groups of muscles and correcting the joints. After a few sessions, the spine gets 90 degree erect. Subsequently a feeling of well-being is felt. When I learned this therapy in Tokyo, it struck me that yoga is a passive technique to induce anatomical symmetry in spinal column. Later studies proved that yoga indeed helps spine to be erect. Therefore, yoga corrects physical asymmetry in the muscutoskeletal structure. Physical symmetry is the cornerstone for health.

Human body has bilateral symmetry. There are two legs, two arms, two eyes, two ears, two lungs, two kidneys etc. However, there is only one stomach, one liver, one spleen, one heart etc. Therefore, some asymmetry results because of internal anatomical asymmetry. This mild asymmetry is augmented by bad posture and bad gait. Unequal wearing of pair of shoes proves this. When the body weight is unequally borne by legs, it results in slight pelvic tilt. The root cause of pathology in many day-to-day illnesses is physical asymmetry. Yoga and yumeiho therapy correct it. In yumeiho, we need a therapist, who works on our body. But yoga is practiced by a person without any help from others. Yoga has to be practiced at least for few months to get satisfactory results. Yumeiho yields results faster than yoga. The rubric of one of my lectures on Yumeiho therapy was 'yoga fast forward'.

The yumeiho centre in Tokyo has a weighing machine with two pedals. When a person stands on it, it records weight of the body separately as shared by each leg. After few sessions of therapy, it shows almost equal weight on both sides. Dr Masayuki has himself devised this weighing machine and proved the efficacy of yumeiho therapy. However, he does not see any relation between yumeiho and yoga. Dr Masayuki has been invited by the Aviation hospital in Moscow, where he treated cosmonauts/astronauts suffering from incurable backache because of their long sojourns in space.

There are hundreds of yoga centers across the world. Yoga has become an exportable commodity. Taichi of China is now competing with yoga. Indian yoga teachers have good market in India and abroad.

Are Ayurveda medicines safe?

It is often overemphasized that ayurveda medicines contain innocuous herbs, with no side effects; instead, they bestow side benefits. Ayurveda is now facing new challenges in India and abroad. In reality, several ayurveda medicines, primarily the herbo-mineral preparations, exported from India are banned in developed countries owing to the presence of heavy metals in unacceptable quantities. The British Museum has exhibited certain ayurveda *rasauṣadas* that are not allowed into Great Britain. The medical bureaucracy in India is not able to screen ayurvedic medicines produced in India for their safety. Physicians of ayurveda believe that *śuddhi* (cleansing) process renders alchemical formulations, containing mercury and other metals, harmless. This is a big myth. Mercury cannot be 'purified' with conventional techniques. There are hundreds of patients in India, who lost their kidneys and liver after prolonged use of alchemical preparations. There is no system to control and contain this bad practice.

People believe that modern medicines contain chemicals as ingredients and ayurveda medicines contain herbals as ingredients. Herbals too are made up of chemicals. Ayurvedic herbs contain certain anti-nutrients like polyphenols. The first herb of ayurveda, *harītaki* (Terminalia chebula), is recommended in several pathologies. It is also known as *rasāyana* i.e. geriatric or life-prolonging substance. However, if used continuously it interferes with absorption of iron from the gut and leads to anemia. *Yashtimadhu* (Glyzerazia glabra) is a highly praised herb used in several pathologies particularly respiratory diseases, arthritis etc. If this herb is used continuously, the patient develops hypertension. On long use of *yashtimadhu* diabetes mellitus too is an impending risk, because this herb contains plant steroids. Hundreds of research papers were published on the toxic effects of herbs on misuse. Ayurveda practitioners are not aware of the real effects of abuse of herbs. These studies are hidden from the public and ignored by the scholars of ayurveda. In fact, many ayurveda physicians do not read the current research result on ayurvedic herbs and alchemical products. The CCIM has to add such related studies to the curriculum of the BAMS course, so that the students of ayurveda become more conscious of the undesirable effects of ayurvedic medicines.

Ayurveda and Public Health in India

The registration of population census in India began under the British administration. The demographics of ancient and medieval India are based on guesswork. The population of India was less than three hundred million a century ago. Now it is more than 1250 million. The population of the Indian subcontinent was fluctuating until the year 1921. Afterwards, population growth was steady and upwards. Demographers call this period as

Great Divide. High infant mortality rate, epidemics and famines were limiting the population until 1921 and ayurveda played no role in improving the situation. The gazetteers of India compiled in 18th and 19th centuries are unequivocal on health statistics. Every year millions die due to cholera, malaria, small pox, plague and other easily preventable diseases. Millions were disfigured due to polio, wars etc. Ayurveda physician accolades ayurveda's role in public health in the yester centuries but the unfortunates will not be rising from their graves to contradict. The life expectance at the beginning of 20th century was around 30. By the middle of the 20th century, it rose to 40 and gradually to 66 now. Not all this happened because of ayurveda.

Maternal Mortality Rate was very high. It is death of women during pregnancy, childbirth or in the 42 days after delivery. India reports now MMR around 250 for 100,000 live births. In 1980, it was 677. It was more than 1000 before any statistics were collected. Absence of family limiting techniques and risks involved in maternal health has halved the lifespan of women. Scientific medicine blessed the women in India.

Easily preventable diseases killed scores of children every day. Childbirth was considered as another incarnation for women. If children die during childbirth or infancy, ayurveda consoled them that the dead infant was not a human being but a devil. *Kaśyapa samhita* crafted a story that justifies that when a devil (*rākṣasa*) occupies womb, the god sends a messenger to kill it. Therefore, a miscarriage is a blessing. It also declares that the sins committed by women are the main cause of her diseases. These dismal historical facts show the ability of ayurveda in public health. The number of children in a family was considered as god-given. Fortunately, the scientific medicine has revolutionized the health status of an average Indian. Now many Indians yearn for *good old days*! It is natural to human psychology to reject the present and long for the past.

The techniques to limit the population too were inadequate in ayurveda. These techniques are not dependable. Therefore, the government of India advocates tubectomy and vasectomy along with pill to limit the size of the family. Ayurveda does not have any say here because the physiological aspects of reproduction are very unscientific in its literature.

The medical statistics in India are intimidating. In India, there are fifteen million blind people, seventy five million physically handicapped (other than blinds), two million suffering from cancer, 2.4 million from HIV, thirty million living with diabetes mellitus and millions running the risk of heart attack. Every year 0.7 million new cancer cases are registered and 0.3 million die of cancer. Among the HIV cases, 39% are women and 3.5% are children. Out of 15 million visually challenged, three fourths of cases are easily preventable if proper precautions were taken at right time.

These mind-boggling problems could be solved by an efficient administration of medical departments and sanitary wings of the regional and local governments. Improvements in the peoples' health happen by prompt garbage collection and recycling, providing potable water and improvements in public transport. Inadequate public transport in towns and cities forces people to invest in private transport and sedentary lifestyle. Consequently, the proportion of degenerative diseases is on the rise. At the dawn of 21st century, more than half of rural population does not have access to toilets and potable drinking water. If money is spent on sanitation, budget allocation to health will significantly comedown. Ayurveda does not know about closed toilets and recycling garbage. Its concepts and practices on social and preventive medicine are not suitable to modern industrial societies. Untreated river water and water from open wells is not safe. The herbal disinfectants like Strychnos potatorum (*kataka*) are not able to clear water from all impurities.

Health services provided by the government of India to its people are inadequate and irrational; therefore, people flock to charlatans and quacks. The lifestyle and outlook of an average Indian is not yet properly influenced by the fruits of science and technology. The health policy of the government of India is inconsistent. Public health is in the concurrent list, i.e. both the federal government and regional (state) governments have say in the health administration. The regional governments have established public hospitals in all towns and cities. People have right to get free treatment. In practice, only poor and destitute people flock to the government hospitals where the physicians are unwilling to work. The quality of nursing is very poor. Always medicines are in scarce. The physicians and surgeons establish their private clinics and thrive. In big cities, luxurious polyclinics and corporate hospitals serve rich patients round the clock. The insurance component is poorly understood in India. The insurance companies involved in the health insurance smile at you when you pay the premium but unhelpful when you need service.

The regional governments in India run thousands of dispensaries of ayurveda, yunani, homeopathy and siddha systems of medicine across the country. These are aimed at providing basic services to the people. However, these ayurveda, homeo, yunani clinics run by the regional governments are not efficient. The entire budget is usurped by the doctor's salary and little remains for the medicines. The doctors too do not like to reside in the rural areas and infrequently commute.

Ambulance service in India is unprofessional. Vehicles are ill equipped, staff unmotivated, underfinanced and insufficient. The World Health Organization recommends at least one ambulance for 100,000 populations. Several ambulances in India are used by doctors and paramedical staff as commuter vehicles. It is always faster to take a patient to the hospital by private means instead of ambulance due to congestion on the roads and unreliable service.

Many non-governmental organizations, social service organizations organize 'medical camps' from time to time. These medical camps dedicated to serve patients just for a day or two address general health problems and a few special diseases. If the government has a network of first-aid centers, dispensaries, primary health centers and referral hospitals working in tandem, organizing makeshift medical camps would be superfluous. In India, medical camps are organized to attract patients to private clinics or to gain political mileage. There may be some philanthropic physicians, who serve the public, but this culture of organizing medical camps has to be discouraged. Organizing one-day mass vaccination for polio and other diseases is also a similar kind of activity. If hospital services are punctual and people-friendly, no such special camps are needed.

Half a century ago, in 1960s, a medical doctor M.C. Modi, an ophthalmologist, toured entire India and operated on thousands of patients for cataract. He attracted the attention of the government of India and non-governmental organizations. He was seen as champion of eye diseases. He received education in ayurveda and modern medicine. Thousands of ophthalmic medical camps arranged in makeshift places in rural and urban areas were flocked by millions of blind people. The people took him as savior and they thought he could give vision to any blind person. After surgical operations, Dr Modi moved on to other places and the operated patients are left with no postoperative care. Dr Modi always went ahead to meet new patients. No statistics were kept but it is a fact that 70% of the patients have developed post-operative infections and total loss of vision was the result. The media has scarcely reported on the bad fallout of Modi's tour of India. Dr Modi was awarded *padmasri* and *padmabhushan* by the government of India. It is recorded that he operated on more than 600,000 patients for cataract surgeries. Modi's episode reflects the poor status of medical service in India half a century ago. Now the picture has not changed much. Organizing medical camps is a sign of dysfunctional medical establishment. Ayurveda physicians love organizing ayurveda medical camps to propagate ayurveda. Ayurveda does not need propagation. If ayurveda physicians stick to their duty, medical ethics and fair-deal in their business, ayurveda will be glorified.

Physician is equated with god in the tradition of India. There were very few instances of punishing erring physicians. Therefore, accountability is less than what it should be. The government has to contain certain unethical practices of both ayurveda and general physicians. Some institutionally qualified ayurveda physicians prescribe medicines to select sex of the unborn baby, curing HIV, cancer and other incurable diseases. Ayurveda classified certain diseases (ex: juvenile diabetes) as incurable, then how and why ayurveda physicians allure patients in such cases? Deceiving patients is a common practice in all the systems of medicine but patients willingly come to ayurveda physicians expecting magic therapies.

Physicians of ayurveda are ignorant of their past and try to convince us that in the past everything was perfect. They assert that ayurveda is scientific but it has lost its glory owing to the rise of modernity. However, they don't realize that if ayurveda could cater to the needs of the people in all situations, western medicine could not have taken shape in the past five centuries.

Out of Balance

The Botanical Survey of India recently prioritized 359 wild medicinal plant species and assessed their availability. The news is disappointing. Of the 359 species, 335 were categorized as critically endangered, endangered, and vulnerable or near threatened. Many important herbs like pepper and myrobalans are in great demand in food and chemical industries, therefore, their availability can be protected. Some herbs which are used in ayurveda (ex: *tālisa* – Abies webbiana) are endangered. Therefore, several substitutes (Taxus baccata for *tālisa*) are used.

Ayurveda recommends the meat of different animals, birds, and lizards in different seasons and diseases. Following these recommendations is mostly illegal today. Therefore, these prescriptions amount to violation of Wildlife Act. In these formulations, several prohibited animal derivatives were recommended like gall stones of tiger, meat of peacock, semen of crocodile etc. As such, most of these prescriptions are outdated and impractical today. However, certain formulations recommended by ayurveda, which were developed by empirical methods, are useful. The range of flora and fauna dealt in the literature of ayurveda is very small of the available biological diversity of the nature. The United Nations Environment Program has estimated the total number of species in the world as 8.7 million and the number of floral and faunal species dealt by ayurveda is around one thousand only!

It is a common conception that ayurveda has discovered valuable herbs in nature useful in food and medicine. Unfortunately, this is not true. Most of the herbs used in ayurveda are much older than ayurveda itself. Pepper (*Piper longum*) was discovered in nature by the tribes of Kerala at least 8000 years ago, even before the Vedic age. Similarly, zinger, turmeric, tamarind etc were discovered in nature long before Caraka or Suśruta could become physicians. Now, the scholars of ayurveda have to realize the real potential of their erudition.

Mahatma Gandhi on Ayurveda

It is interesting to know the views of Mahatma Gandhi, father of the nation, on ayurveda. Gandhi has not come out of religion to become a politician. He is seen as a pious Hindu. His Complete Works allude to ayurveda at several places. He says 'traditional medicines like ayurveda and yunani, had unlike western science, maintained a relation between science and religion, body and soul, but had not inculcated the spirit of research that fired modern science and gave it contemporary relevance.' In 1921, inaugurating thc Tibbia College at Delhi, Gandhi expounded his views on modern and traditional medicine. He lauded the spirit of inquiry of the modern scientists: I would like to pay my humble tribute to the spirit of research that fires the modern scientists. My quarrel is not against that spirit. My complaint is against the direction that the spirit had taken. It has chiefly concerned itself with the exploration of laws and methods conducing to the merely material advancement of its clientele. But I have nothing but praise for the zeal, industry and sacrifice that have animated the modern scientists in the pursuit after truth. I regret to have to record my opinion based on considerable experience that our *hakims* and *vaids* (yunani and ayurvedic practitioners) do not exhibit that spirit in any mentionable degree. They follow without question formulas. They carry on little investigation. The condition of indigenous medicine is truly deplorable. Not having kept abreast of modern research, their profession has fallen largely into disrepute. I am hoping that this college will try to remedy this grave defect and restore ayurvedic and yunani medical sciences to its pristine glory.

In 1925, Mahatma Gandhi addressed audience at the Ayurvedic Pharmacy, Madras and later, in the same year, he inaugurated Aṣṭānga Ayurvedic Vidyalaya at Calcutta. On both these occasions, he expressed his criticism on ayurvedic physicians. He was pained by large-scale advertisements primarily of ayurvedic tonics as sexual stimulants, ample proof that ayurvedic physicians were merely trying to capitalize on past glories of ayurveda for the market without any genuine research. He bemoaned the fact that there was no association of ayurvedic physicians that protested against these immoral business and unethical practices. Testifying to the spirit of the western physicians, he remarked that despite his strong views on modern medicine one thing that it had in its favor was humility of its practitioners and its research. He wished that this spirit would fire the ayurvedic physicians too. Ayurveda's lost glory could only be recovered if the *vaids* acquired honesty of purpose and pursued the research spirit of the west.

Gandhi's controversial speech at Calcutta evoked a letter from Kaviraj Gananath Sen, a senior practitioner, asking that Gandhi clarify his stand on ayurveda. In his response, Gandhi repeated that many ayurvedic practitioners were mere quacks pretending to know much more than they actually did and arrogating to themselves infallibility and ability to cure all diseases. Instead of studying ayurvedic system and wresting from it secrets which appeared to be completely hidden from the world, they imputed to ayurveda omnipotence making it a stagnant system instead of a gloriously progressive science. His criticism was about lack of humility and complacency of professors of ayurveda and not the discipline itself. He remarked provocatively that: 'I know of not a single discovery or invention of any importance on the part of ayurvedic physicians as against a brilliant array of discoveries and inventions which western physicians and surgeons boast'. Elaborating his position, as some *vaids* were not satisfied with Gandhi's response, Gandhi added: I do like everything that is ancient and noble, but I utterly dislike a parody of it. And I must respectfully refuse to believe that ancient books are the last word on the matters treated in them. As a wise heir to the ancients, I am desirous of adding to and enriching the legacy inherited by us.

Glossary of Ayurvedic Terms

abhiṣeka pouring of sacred liquids on to the idol

abhraka mica

agniveṣa author of Carakasamhita, student of Ātreya

aharana extracting

ākāṣ space element

anga organ, branch

ap water element

apasmāra epilepsy

ariṣṭa a pharmaceutical preparation with self generated alcohol

āsavaa pharmaceutical preparation with self generated alcohol

aṣṭasthānaparīkṣa examination of eight locations, a diagnostic technique

asthi bone

aśva horse

ātmasoul

Ātreya guru of Aginveśa, author of Carakasamhita

auṣada medicine

ayurveda traditional Indian system of medicine

bālaroga diseases of the children

bhaiṣajyakalpana formulation of medicines

bhasma cinder

bhedana incision

bhiṣak physician

bhutavidya demonology

cala mobile

chedana cutting
Dhanvantari god of ayurveda, propounded of surgical school of medicine
dhāra pouring medicated oil on the forehead (Keraliya treatments)
dhātu constituent factor
dhātuvāda part of alchemy to manufacture gold from inferior metals.
Digambara one of the two traditions of Jainism
drava liquid
eṣana exploring/probing
gandhaka sulphur
gauripāṣanam arsenic penta-sulphide
grahacikitsa demonology
griṣma summer season
guru heavy
hemanta winter season
hima cold
jnānendriya sensory organ
kanda part, chapter
kandagam sulphur
kapha one of the three humors
karmendriya motor organ
kaṭhina hard
kāyacikitsa internal medicine
khara rough
kumkum vermilion
laghu light, weightless
lavaṇa salt
lekhana scrapping
majja bone-marrow

makaradhvaja a pharmaceutical preparation of ayurveda
mala excreta, feces, impurity
māmsa muscular tissue, one of the constituents of the human body.
manas mind
manda slow
meda fat
medha intellect
mṛdu soft
mutra urine
nāḍi (radial) pulse
navara kizzi one of the Kerala ayurveda treatments done with new rice.
pancakarma five modalities of treatment
pārada quick silver, mercury
picchila slimy
pita bluish
pitta one of the three humors
pizichchil one of the Kerala treatments of *panchakarma*.
prasuti midwifery
pravṛt ṛtu season between the summer and monsoon.
prithvi earth, one of the five elements that constitute the universe
puruṣa human being
rajas menstrual blood
rajo valor
rakta blood, red
rasa taste, mercury, one of the constituent factor of the body

rasaśāstra alchemy
rasāyana geriatrics
ratna jewel
rukṣa dry
rupa appearance
śabda sound
śalākya surgery of ear, nose, throat, dentistry and head diseases.
śalya general surgery
sāndra solid
śarad post-monsoon season with clear moon
saram flowing
sarpavidya toxicology
sarvaśalya general surgery
saṣṭika dhānya cereals that grow in sixty days
satva inner strength, good sense
siddha sage, system of medicine in extreme south of India
śilājit black bitumen
śiśira season after the monsoon season, fall
sita cold
sivana suturing
slakṣṇa smooth
sloka hymn
snigdha unctuous
sthira stable
sthula gross
striroga diseases of women
sukra semen
sukṣma subtle
śvasthavritha social and preventive medicine
śvetambara one of the two Jaina traditions
tamas dark
teja fire element

tikshna quick, sharp
unmāda psychological disorder (madness)
vajapeya ritual of sacrifice for bountiful crop; vaja is rice, peya is drink.

Vājikaraṇa aphrodisialogy

varṣa monsoon season (rainy)

vasantha spring season
vāta (wind) a humor, which regulates bodily functions.
vāyu air element
vellai paṣanam white arsenic
viram mercuric chloride

viṣa poison

viṣada non-slimy

visrāvanaooze out
vyadhana making holes
yunani system of medicine popular among Muslims.

www.ingramcontent.com/pod-product-compliance
Lightning Source LLC
Chambersburg PA
CBHW050438290526
45786CB00006B/2079
* 9 7 8 1 5 2 0 2 7 2 5 8 0 *